TOP TRAILS

Shenandoah National Park

50 MUST-DO HIKES FOR EVERYONE

SECOND EDITION

Johnny Molloy

 WILDERNESS PRESS . . . *on the trail since 1967*

Top Trails Shenandoah National Park: 50 Must-Do Hikes for Everyone

Copyright © 2018 by Johnny Molloy
Second edition, third printing 2022

Project editor: Ritchey Halphen
Photos: Copyright © 2018 by Johnny Molloy, except where noted
Cartography: Scott McGrew and Johnny Molloy
Cover and interior design: Frances Baca
Copyeditor: Erin Mahoney
Proofreaders: Laura Franck, Scott Alexander Jones
Indexer: Meghan Miller Brawley/Potomac Indexing

Library of Congress Cataloging-in-Publication Data

Names: Molloy, Johnny, 1961– author.
Title: Top trails Shenandoah National Park : must-do hikes for everyone / written by
    Johnny Molloy.
Description: Second edition. | Birmingham, AL : Wilderness Press, 2018. | Series: Top trails |
    Includes index.
Identifiers: LCCN 2017058780 | ISBN 978-0-89997-878-9 (pbk.) | ISBN 978-0-89997-879-6
    (ebook)
Subjects: LCSH: Hiking—Virginia—Shenandoah National Park—Guidebooks. | Trails—
    Virginia—Shenandoah National Park—Guidebooks. | Shenandoah National Park
    (Va.)—Guidebooks.
Classification: LCC GV199.42.V82 S4847 2018 | DDC 796.5109755—dc23
    LC record available at lccn.loc.gov/2017058780

Manufactured in the United States of America

WILDERNESS PRESS
An imprint of AdventureKEEN
2204 First Ave. S., Ste. 102
Birmingham, AL 35233
800-678-7006; fax 877-374-9016

Visit wildernesspress.com for a complete listing of our books and for ordering information. Contact us at our website, at facebook.com/wildernesspress1967, or at twitter.com/wilderness 1967 with questions or comments. To find out more about who we are and what we're doing, visit blog.wildernesspress.com.

Cover photo: High fall color in Shenandoah National Park; Christian Hinkle/Shutterstock

SAFETY NOTICE Although Wilderness Press and Johnny Molloy have made every attempt to ensure that the information in this book is accurate at press time, they are not responsible for any loss, damage, injury, or inconvenience that may occur to anyone while using this book. You are responsible for your own safety and health while in the wilderness. The fact that a trail is described in this book does not mean that it will be safe for you. Be aware that trail conditions can change from day to day. Always check local conditions, know your own limitations, and consult a map.

The Top Trails Series

Wilderness Press

When Wilderness Press published *Sierra North* in 1967, no other trail guide like it existed for the Sierra backcountry. The first run of 2,800 copies sold out in less than two months, and its success heralded the beginning of Wilderness Press. Since we were founded more than 50 years ago, we have expanded our territories to cover California, Alaska, Hawaii, the US Southwest, the Pacific Northwest, New England, Canada, and the Southeast, including Virginia's Shenandoah National Park.

Wilderness Press continues to publish comprehensive, accurate, and readable outdoor books. Hikers, backpackers, kayakers, skiers, snowshoers, climbers, cyclists, and trail runners rely on Wilderness Press for accurate outdoor adventure information.

Top Trails

In its Top Trails guides, Wilderness Press has paid special attention to organization so that you can find the perfect hike each and every time. Whether you're looking for a steep trail to test yourself on or a walk in the park, a romantic waterfall or a city view, Top Trails will lead you there.

Each Top Trails guide contains trails for everyone. The trails selected provide a sampling of the best that the region has to offer. These are the "must-do" hikes and walks, with every feature of the area represented.

Every book in the Top Trails series offers the following:

- The Wilderness Press commitment to accuracy and reliability
- Ratings and rankings for each trail
- Distances and approximate times
- Easy-to-follow trail notes
- Map and permit information

Shenandoah National Park Map

TRAIL FEATURES TABLE

Shenandoah National Park Trails

TRAIL NUMBER AND NAME	Page	Difficulty −12345+	Length in Miles	Type	Dayhiking	Backpacking	Child-Friendly	Pets Prohibited	
1. North District									
1 Dickey Ridge Historic Hike	29	2	4.3	↻	🚶			⊗	
2 Compton Peak	35	3	3.2	↗	🚶				
3 Big Devils Stairs Vista	39	3	5.0	↗	🚶	🎒			
4 Sugarloaf Loop	45	3	4.7	↻	🚶	🎒			
5 Overall Run Falls	49	4	6.8	↗	🚶				
6 Little Devils Stairs Loop	55	4	5.4	↻	🚶	🎒			
7 Overall Run Loop	61	5	9.2	↻	🚶	🎒			
8 Heiskell Hollow Loop	67	4	7.2	↻	🚶	🎒			
9 Elkwallow Loop	71	3	5.6	↻	🚶				
10 Piney River Falls	75	4	6.8	↗	🚶	🎒			
11 Knob Mountain and Jeremys Run Loop	81	5	13.1	↻	🚶	🎒			
12 Neighbor Mountain and Jeremys Run Loop	87	5	14.0	↻	🚶	🎒			
13 Thornton River Loop	93	4	7.9	↻	🚶	🎒			
2. Central District									
14 Marys Rock via The Pinnacle	111	3	7.2	↗	🚶				
15 Hazel Falls and Cave	117	3	5.2	↗	🚶		👫		
16 Hazel Country Loop	121	5	16.8	↻	🚶	🎒			
17 Corbin Cabin Hike	127	3	2.8	↗	🚶				
18 Old Rag Loop	131	5	9.1	↻	🚶			⊗	
19 Stony Man Loop	137	3	3.4	↻	🚶			⊗	
20 Robertson Mountain	143	4	6.8	↗	🚶				
21 Falls of Whiteoak Canyon	149	4	5.2	↗	🚶				
22 Cedar Run Falls	155	4	3.4	↗	🚶				
23 Hawksbill Summit	159	2	2.2	↗	🚶				
24 Rose River Falls Loop	163	3	4.0	↻	🚶	🎒			
25 Lewis Spring Falls Loop	169	3	3.3	↻	🚶				

TYPE	DIFFICULTY −12345+ less more	TERRAIN
↻ Loop		△ Summit ▷ Stream
↗ Out-and-Back	USES & ACCESS	▲ Ridgeline ◣ Waterfall
	🚶 Day Hiking 👫 Child-Friendly	
	🎒 Backpacking ⊗ Pets Prohibited	

TRAIL FEATURES TABLE

#	Summit	Ridgeline	Stream	Waterfall	Autumn Colors	Wildflowers	Wildlife	Old-Growth	Great Views	Camping	Swimming	Secluded	Steep	Historical Interest	Geological Interest
1		●			●				●					●	
2	●	●			●				●						●
3		●	●		●	●			●						
4		●	●		●		●		●						●
5		●	●	●	●	●	●		●	●					●
6		●	●		●	●			●					●	●
7		●	●	●	●		●		●	●	●	●	●	●	●
8		●	●		●	●	●			●		●		●	
9		●	●		●	●	●			●		●			
10		●	●	●	●	●						●			
11	●	●	●	●	●		●		●		●	●	●		●
12	●	●	●	●	●	●			●		●	●	●		
13	●	●	●	●	●	●	●					●		●	
14		●			●				●						●
15		●	●	●	●	●									●
16		●	●		●	●			●			●	●	●	●
17		●	●		●	●								●	
18	●	●	●		●	●			●						●
19	●	●			●	●			●					●	●
20	●	●	●		●				●						
21			●	●		●			●				●		
22			●	●	●	●							●		●
23	●				●				●						
24			●	●	●									●	●
25	●	●	●	●	●	●			●						●

NATURE
- Autumn Colors
- Wildflowers
- Wildlife
- Old-Growth Forest

FEATURES
- Great Views
- Camping
- Swimming
- Secluded
- Steep
- Historical Interest
- Geological Interest

TRAIL FEATURES TABLE

Shenandoah National Park Trails

TRAIL NUMBER AND NAME	Page	Difficulty −1 2 3 4 5 +	Length in Miles	Type	Day hiking	Backpacking	Child-Friendly	Pets Prohibited
2. Central District (continued)								
26 Hazeltop and Rapidan Camp Loop	175	4	7.2	↻	🚶	🎒		
27 Staunton River Loop	181	5	18.6	↻	🚶	🎒		
28 Bear Church Rock via Staunton River	187	5	7.6	↗	🚶	🎒		
29 Bear Church Rock from Bootens Gap	193	4	9.4	↗	🚶			
30 Conway River Loop	197	5	12.0	↻	🚶	🎒		⊗
31 Bearfence Mountain Rock Scramble	205	3	1.1	↻	🚶			⊗
32 Pocosin Mission	209	2	2.0	↗	🚶		👫	
33 South River Falls Loop	213	3	4.5	↻	🚶			
3. South District								
34 Hightop	231	3	3.2	↗	🚶	🎒		
35 Rocky Mount Loop	235	5	9.8	↻	🚶	🎒		
36 Rocky Mountain Loop	241	5	9.5	↻	🚶	🎒		
37 Loft Mountain Loop	247	2	2.9	↻	🚶			⊗
38 Patterson Ridge Loop	251	5	9.7	↻	🚶	🎒		
39 Big Run Loop	257	3	5.8	↻	🚶			
40 Rockytop and Big Run Loop	263	5	13.3	↻	🚶	🎒		
41 Austin Mountain and Madison Run Loop	269	4	8.8	↻	🚶	🎒		
42 Falls Loop from Browns Gap	275	4	7.0	↻	🚶	🎒		
43 Trayfoot Mountain Loop	279	5	20.7	↻	🚶	🎒		
44 Furnace Mountain via Blackrock	287	3	6.8	↗	🚶	🎒		
45 Blackrock Loop	293	1	1.1	↻	🚶		👫	
46 Big Branch Falls via Moormans River	297	4	7.6	↗	🚶	🎒		
47 Moormans River Loop	301	5	18.3	↻	🚶	🎒		
48 Chimney Rock	305	2	3.2	↗	🚶	🎒		
49 Turk Branch Loop	315	4	7.5	↻	🚶	🎒		
50 Turk Mountain	321	2	2.4	↗	🚶			

TYPE	DIFFICULTY −1 2 3 4 5 + less more	TERRAIN
↻ Loop		△ Summit ▷ Stream
↗ Out-and-Back	USES & ACCESS	▲ Ridgeline ▮ Waterfall
	🚶 Day Hiking 👫 Child-Friendly	
	🎒 Backpacking ⊗ Pets Prohibited	

TRAIL FEATURES TABLE

#	Summit	Ridgeline	Stream	Waterfall	Autumn Colors	Wildflowers	Wildlife	Old-Growth	Great Views	Camping	Swimming	Secluded	Steep	Historical Interest	Geological Interest
26	✓	✓	✓	✓	✓	✓	✓		✓					✓	
27		✓	✓	✓	✓				✓	✓	✓	✓		✓	✓
28		✓	✓	✓	✓	✓			✓		✓	✓			
29		✓			✓				✓			✓		✓	✓
30		✓	✓	✓	✓	✓		✓	✓					✓	✓
31		✓			✓										✓
32		✓			✓	✓		✓	✓					✓	
33			✓	✓	✓	✓									✓
34	✓				✓	✓			✓						✓
35	✓	✓	✓		✓	✓			✓					✓	✓
36		✓	✓	✓	✓				✓		✓		✓		✓
37		✓			✓	✓			✓	✓					✓
38		✓	✓		✓	✓			✓	✓	✓	✓			
39		✓	✓		✓	✓			✓					✓	✓
40		✓	✓		✓				✓		✓	✓	✓	✓	
41		✓	✓		✓	✓			✓					✓	
42		✓	✓	✓	✓	✓		✓						✓	✓
43	✓	✓	✓		✓	✓	✓		✓		✓	✓		✓	✓
44	✓	✓			✓				✓			✓			✓
45	✓	✓			✓				✓						✓
46			✓	✓	✓	✓					✓	✓			
47		✓	✓	✓	✓	✓	✓		✓		✓	✓		✓	
48		✓			✓				✓						✓
49		✓	✓	✓	✓	✓						✓		✓	
50		✓	✓	✓	✓	✓						✓		✓	✓

Column groups: TERRAIN (Summit, Ridgeline, Stream, Waterfall) · NATURE (Autumn Colors, Wildflowers, Wildlife, Old-Growth) · OTHER (Great Views, Camping, Swimming, Secluded, Steep, Historical Interest, Geological Interest)

NATURE
- Autumn Colors
- Wildflowers
- Wildlife
- Old-Growth Forest

FEATURES
- Great Views
- Camping
- Swimming
- Secluded
- Steep
- Historical Interest
- Geological Interest

Contents

Opposite: *Piney River Falls (Trail 10, page 75) fans out over a rock face before splashing into a pool.*

CHAPTER 1
North District

CHAPTER 2
Central District

CHAPTER 3
South District

Using Top Trails

Organization of Top Trails

Top Trails is designed to make identifying the perfect trail easy and enjoyable, and to make every outing a success and a pleasure. With this book you'll find it's a snap to find the right trail, whether you're planning a major hike or just a sociable stroll with friends.

The Region

Each Top Trails guide begins with the overview map (pages iv–v), displaying the entire area covered by this guide and providing an overview of the geography. The map is clearly marked to show which area is covered by each chapter.

After the overview map comes the master trails table (pages vi–ix), which lists every trail covered in the guide. Here you'll find a concise description, basic information, and highlighted features, all indispensable when planning an outing. A quick reading of the regional map and trails table will give you a good overview of the entire region covered by the book.

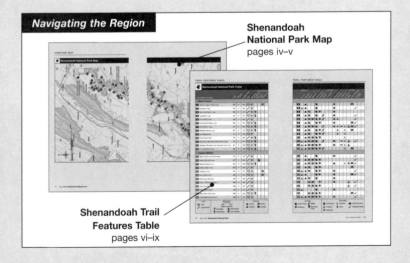

Navigating the Region

Shenandoah
National Park Map
pages iv–v

Shenandoah Trail
Features Table
pages vi–ix

The Areas

The region covered in each book is divided into areas, with each chapter corresponding to one area in the region. Each area chapter introduction starts with information to help you choose and enjoy a trail every time out. Use the table of contents or the regional map to identify an area of interest, and then turn to the area chapter to find the following:

- An overview of the area, including park and permit information
- An area map showing all trail locations
- A trail features table providing trail-by-trail details
- Trail summaries highlighting each trail's specific features

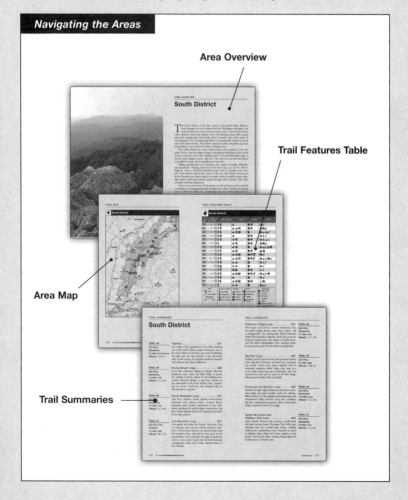

Navigating the Areas

Area Overview

Trail Features Table

Area Map

Trail Summaries

The Trails

The basic building block of the Top Trails guide is the trail entry. Each one is laid out to make finding and following the trail as simple as possible, with all pertinent information presented in this easy-to-follow format:

- A detailed trail map
- Trail descriptors covering difficulty, length, and other essential data
- A written trail description
- Trail milestones providing easy-to-follow, turn-by-turn trail directions

Some trail descriptions offer additional information:

- An elevation profile
- Trail options
- Trail highlights

In the margins of the trail entries, keep your eyes open for graphic icons that signal features mentioned in the text.

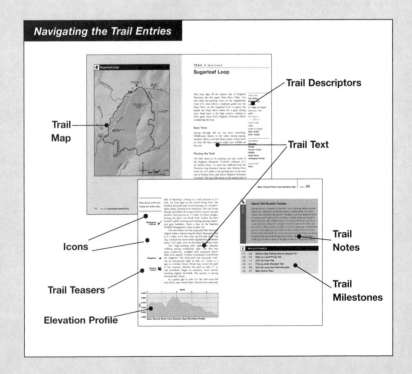

Choosing a Trail

Top Trails provides several different ways of choosing a trail, all presented in easy-to-read tables, charts, and maps.

Location

If you know in general where you want to go, Top Trails makes it easy to find the right trail in the right place. Each chapter begins with a large-scale map showing the starting point of every trail in that area.

Features

This guide describes the Top Trails of Shenandoah National Park, and each trail is chosen because it offers one or more features that make it appealing. Using the trail descriptions, summaries, and tables, you can quickly examine all the trails for the features they offer or seek a particular feature among the list of trails.

Best Time

Time of year and current conditions can be important factors in selecting the best trail. For example, an exposed low-elevation trail may be a riot of color in early spring but an oven-baked taste of hell in midsummer. Wherever relevant, Top Trails identifies the best and worst conditions for the trails you plan to hike.

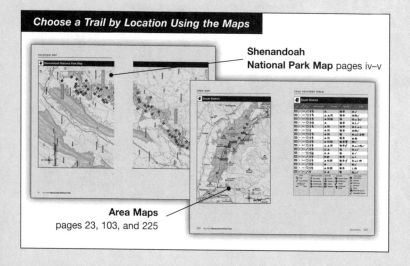

Choose a Trail by Location Using the Maps

Shenandoah National Park Map pages iv–v

Area Maps pages 23, 103, and 225

Difficulty

Every trail has an overall difficulty rating on a scale of 1–5, which takes into consideration length, elevation change, exposure, trail quality, etc., to create one (admittedly subjective) rating.

The ratings assume you are an able-bodied adult in reasonably good shape, using the trail for hiking. The ratings also assume normal weather conditions—clear and dry.

Readers should make an honest assessment of their own abilities and adjust time estimates accordingly. Also, rain, snow, heat, wind, and poor visibility can all affect your pace on even the easiest of trails.

The Elevation Factor

Cumulative Elevation Gain and Loss

The at-a-glance info in the margin of each Top Trails entry includes a pair of numbers labeled **Vertical Feet**. The numbers represent the *total gain* and/or *total loss of altitude* as you negotiate the trail's ascents and descents between the beginning and ending points of the hike.

For hikes that start and end at the same spot—that is, a loop or an out-and-back trail—the elevation gain matches the elevation loss because you're essentially retracing your route. (Exceptions—which are reflected

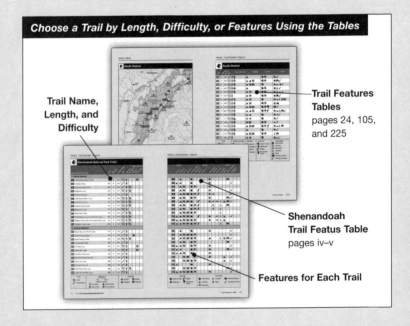

Choose a Trail by Length, Difficulty, or Features Using the Tables

Trail Name, Length, and Difficulty

Trail Features Tables
pages 24, 105, and 225

Shenandoah Trail Featus Table
pages iv–v

Features for Each Trail

Map Legend

Featured trail	———————			
Alternate trail	··················			
Appalachian Trail	---------◇---------			
Freeway	⬭⬭⬭⬭⬭⬭⬭⬭		Water body	
Major road	⬭⬭⬭⬭⬭⬭⬭⬭		River/creek	～～～
Minor road	⬭⬭⬭⬭⬭⬭⬭⬭		Intermittent stream	–·–·–·–
Unpaved road	================		Park boundary	

Amphitheater	♨	Point of interest	●
Campground	▲	Radio tower	📡
Cemetery	✝	Ranger station	🏠
Equestrian trail	🐎	Rapids/cascades	〰
Footbridge	✕	Restroom	🚻
Gate	✐	Shelter	⊏
Marsh area	⚶	Spring	○
Milepost	12.4	Swimming access	🏊
Mine site	✕	Tower	🗼
Parking area	P	Trailhead and parking	🚶
Peak	▲	Vista point	🔭
Picnic area	⛱	Waterfall	∥

Top Trails Difficulty Ratings

1 A short trail, generally level, that can be completed in 1 hour
  or less.

2 A route of 1–3 miles, with some ups and downs, that can be
  completed in 1–2 hours.

3 A longer route, up to 5 miles, with some uphill and/or
  downhill sections.

4 A long or steep route—perhaps more than 5 miles or with
  climbs of more than 1,000 vertical feet.

5 The most demanding route: both long and steep and more
  than 5 miles long, with climbs of more than 1,000 vertical feet.

in the numbers—might include, for instance, an optional spur that you take outbound but not inbound.)

With a point-to-point, or one-way, route, the elevation gain and loss will most likely differ. In either case, for matching or differing figures, the author provides both sets of numbers, preceded by a plus or minus sign.

Example: Picture an out-and-back trail that starts at 1,500', climbs to 1,700', descends to 1,500', and climbs to 2,800' at the turnaround point. The hiker reverses course and descends 1,300', climbs 200', and descends 200'. Coming and going, the elevation gain and elevation loss each total 1,300', represented as **Vertical Feet: +1,300'/–1,300'** for this hike. If, however, at that 2,800' turnaround point, the hiker has arranged for a shuttle and this is a point-to-point hike, then the cumulative elevation change would be +1,500'/–200'.

Elevation Profile

To show these incremental ups and downs, each Top Trails entry includes an elevation profile. This graphic element provides a visual guide to the rises and falls you can expect along the hike. For example, one trail's cumulative elevation may total +1,300'/–1,300', and the elevation profile shows that the gain and loss occur as you climb and descend only one peak. Another trail's cumulative elevation may be identical (that is, +1,300'/–1,300'), but its elevation profile may reveal many small rises and falls all along the trail to reach that total.

Thus, you'll want to review both the cumulative elevation number(s) and the elevation profile to know whether your climbs and descents will be many small ones or a few long and arduous ones.

Introduction to Shenandoah National Park

Shenandoah National Park is a scenic mountain haven of the Eastern Seaboard, a glittering jewel in the Appalachian range. What makes Shenandoah so special? First, consider panoramic views from overlooks scattered along lofty Skyline Drive, which runs the length of this 300-square-mile sanctuary. Beyond Skyline Drive lies another Shenandoah, where bears furtively roam the hollows and brook trout ply the tumbling streams. Quartz, granite, and greenstone outcrops jut above the diverse forest, allowing far-flung views of the Blue Ridge and surrounding Shenandoah Valley.

You must reach this other Shenandoah, beyond Skyline Drive, by foot. The rewards increase with every footfall beneath the stately oaks of the ridgetops and in the deep canyons where waterfalls roar among old-growth trees spared by the logger's axe. In some places your footsteps lead past what once were pioneer farms. These homesites reveal another era of Shenandoah. This rich cultural history found settlers squeezed into the narrow valleys and apple orchards lining grassy fields atop the ridges, where lives were made in the craggy Appalachian highlands.

This meld of natural and cultural history is fitting in Virginia, where so much of this country's story has been played out, from the battles of the American Revolution and Civil War to battles in Congress regarding the very establishment of this park. Since its inception, Shenandoah National Park has also seen the cutting down and reforestation of the park, the building of Skyline Drive, the return of the deer and bears, and the invasion of exotic pests that threaten the mountain trees. It has seen park facilities built, fall to disrepair, and become new again. And through it all, Shenandoah has shone.

Shenandoah National Park continues to undergo changes. And in nature, changes come quickly—as in the Rocky Mount Fire of 2016, the prescribed burns to preserve Big Meadows, or the thousand-year flood of 1995. But changes also come slowly, such as the recovery from the gypsy moth infestation of the 1990s and the demise of the hemlock at the hands of the hemlock woolly adelgid in the early 2000s. In any case, Shenandoah continues to display its mountain beauty and come back better than ever. Air quality continues to improve since a low point in the 1970s, allowing for more extensive views year-round.

Choosing Shenandoah as a place to spend your free time is a wise decision. And yet the park can be intimidating, especially for the first-time visitor. Not only are there hundreds of miles of trails running like veins down and along a narrow mountain spine, but with millions of guests annually, Shenandoah National Park is a heavily visited destination—quite intimidating indeed. This book was conceived to make the backcountry majesty of Shenandoah more accessible to visitors.

With this national park's many trails and people, discovering its beauty and solitude can be a hit-or-miss proposition. Where are the spectacular vistas? Where are the waterfalls and the old settlers' homesites? Where can I find solitude? Leaving it all to chance doesn't offer good odds for an all-too-brief vacation from the rat race. Weeks spent daydreaming of a fleeting slice of freedom could culminate in a 3-hour driving marathon or a noisy walk up a crowded trail. Fortunately, with this book and a little bit of planning and forethought, you can make the most of your national park experience.

May this book be as beneficial to your Shenandoah experience as it has been to mine. I've been hiking Shenandoah since the 1980s and have had a Shenandoah guide in print since 1998, with multiple updated and improved editions, including the one in your hand. Penning and then updating this guide for Wilderness Press gave me the chance to rehike all the trails and write another guide to what I think is one of the most beautiful places in the United States. You'll find this very accessible book a marked improvement over my previous Shenandoah guides, and further improved for this latest edition.

This guide presents 50 hikes with plenty of variety. The majority steer you toward the most scenic areas, giving you the opportunity to enjoy your time on the trail instead of behind someone else's car. Most hikes seek solitude to maximize your Shenandoah experience, but as the subtitle suggests, there are some must-do popular hikes. Consequently, a few hikes traverse popular and potentially crowded areas. Each hike lists a Best Time that will help you manage the trails to your advantage.

Classic hikes, such as Old Rag and the falls of Whiteoak Canyon, along with seldom-visited gems, such as Piney River Falls and Furnace Mountain, are represented. Though the latter are not as well known, they offer more solitude than and equally scenic sights as the more popular hikes so that you can discover Shenandoah on your own terms.

Often, park sightseers pick a hike randomly without knowing where it will lead, or they follow the crowds wherever they go. Many times, I've been stopped with the question, "What's down this trail?" Choosing a hike at random in Shenandoah, where many trails drop steeply off the Blue Ridge, may result in a disappointing trip followed by a rigorous return to the car with little reward to show for your effort. This guide provides easy means to find hikes to suit your desires.

This book features two types of hikes: out-and-back and loop. Out-and-back hikes lead to a particularly rewarding destination and return you to the start on the same trail. The return trip allows you to see everything from the opposite vantage point. You may notice more minute trailside features the second go-round. Returning at a different time of day may give the same trail a surprisingly different character. For some hikers, though, returning on the same trail simply isn't enjoyable when 500 additional miles of Shenandoah trails await them. For these hikers, the loops provide a great alternative.

Day hiking is the best and most popular way to break into the Shenandoah wilderness—Shenandoah, in fact, is one of the finest day-hiking parks in our country. But those with the inclination to see the mountain cycle from day to night and back again can enjoy many of these hikes, too. Some of the latest hike additions are longer loops ideal for backpacking, but if you plan to hike overnight, you should be aware of the park's backcountry-camping regulations (see page 6) and practice Leave No Trace wilderness use (see "Trail Etiquette," page 16).

When you tour Shenandoah, you may find it tempting to remain in your car and enjoy the sights along Skyline Drive. While auto touring allows an overview of the park, vehicles create a barrier between you and the wilderness beyond. "Windshield tourists" hoping to observe wildlife often end up observing only the cars around them. While overlooks avail easy views, the hassle of driving, the drone of the car engine, and the lack of effort in reaching the views can make them less than inspirational.

Shenandoah is great for hiking. The wilderness experience can unleash your mind and body, allowing you to relax and find peace and quiet. It also enables you to grasp beauty and splendor: a white-quartz outcrop with a window overlooking the patchwork valley below, a bobcat disappearing into a laurel thicket, or a snow-covered clearing marking an old homestead. On these protected lands, you can let your mind roam where it pleases, something you simply can't do in a climate-controlled automobile. Hiking is the best way to enjoy this special preserve, so get out and enjoy Shenandoah!

Shenandoah National Park: An Overview

Getting There and Getting Around

Bounded by I-66 to the north and I-64 to the south, Shenandoah National Park is located in northwestern Virginia, about 70 miles west of Washington, DC; 93 miles west of Richmond; and 24 miles west of Charlottesville.

To reach the **Front Royal** entrance at the northern end of the park, take Exit 6 off of I-66 onto US 340/US 522, heading south through the town of Front Royal. Drive 4.2 miles and turn left (south) onto Skyline Drive, the main thoroughfare through the park. **GPS: N38° 54.344' W78° 11.917'.**

To reach the **Rockfish Gap** entrance at the southern end of the park, take Exit 99 off of westbound I-64 onto US 250, follow the signs 0.3 mile south and east to Skyline Drive, and turn left (north) to enter the park. **GPS: N38° 02.026' W78° 51.541'.**

The **Thornton Gap** entrance is just north of Lee Highway/US 211, inside the northern third of the park (**GPS: N38° 39.658' W78° 19.246'**), and the **Swift Run Gap** entrance is just off Spotswood Trail/US 33, on the park's western edge (**GPS: N38° 21.970' W78° 34.732'**). The Swift Run Gap entrance is also the only one with a physical address: **22591 Spotswood Trail, Elkton, VA 22827.**

For detailed driving directions, along with Google maps that you can use to create your own directions, visit nps.gov/shen/planyourvisit/directions.htm.

The park is technically open year-round, although certain facilities are open only seasonally. Entrance fees vary depending on the type of vehicle; visitors under age 16 are admitted free. Check before you go for the latest information on operating hours and admission prices: 540-999-3500, nps.gov/shen/planyourvisit.

Skyline Drive bisects the park from north to south along its 105-mile length. Mileposts along the way mark important landmarks; all park maps and informational materials use these mileposts as a reference. A driving map of the entire park is available at nps.gov/shen/planyourvisit/upload/whole_park.pdf. *Note that the speed limit on Skyline Drive is 35 miles per hour.*

Lodging

Hotel-style accommodations are available at **Skyland Resort** (milepost 41.7) and **Big Meadows Lodge** (milepost 51.2). **Lewis Mountain Cabins** (milepost 57.5) are more rustic than the two lodges (which also offer dining and entertainment) but more luxurious than the backcountry cabins maintained by the **Potomac Appalachian Trail Club** (see next page). For reservations and additional information, call 877-247-9261 or visit www.goshenandoah.com/lodging.

Waysides

A unique Shenandoah amenity, a *wayside* is a combination convenience store, camping-supply store, restaurant, and gift shop. The park has three waysides: the **Elkwallow Wayside** at milepost 24.1, the **Big Meadows Wayside** at milepost 51.2 (which also sells gasoline), and the **Loft Mountain Wayside** at milepost 79.5. For hours and additional information, visit www.goshenandoah.com/dining/food-groceries.

Camping

Developed (frontcountry) camping is available at the park's five official campgrounds. See nps.gov/shen/planyourvisit/campgrounds.htm for details. Stay limits are 14 consecutive nights in season and 30 consecutive nights in the off-season.

Backpackers must obtain a free backcountry permit to camp overnight in the wilds of Shenandoah. Permits can be obtained at the following places during business hours, starting at the north end of the park:

Front Royal Entrance Station, milepost 0.6 on Skyline Drive

Dickey Ridge Visitor Center, milepost 4.6 on Skyline Drive

Panorama, milepost 31.6 on Skyline Drive

Old Rag Fee Station, off Nethers Road/VA 600 on the eastern edge of the park (GPS: N38° 34.297' W78° 17.346')

Big Meadows, milepost 51.2 on Skyline Drive

Swift Run Gap Entrance Station, milepost 65.7 on Skyline Drive

Loft Mountain Information Station, milepost 79.5 on Skyline Drive

Rockfish Gap Entrance Station, milepost 104.9 on Skyline Drive

Permits for Appalachian Trail long-distance hikers are available by self-registration on the AT where it enters Shenandoah National Park from both the north and the south.

You can also obtain a backcountry camping permit by mail when you plan your trip at least two weeks in advance by contacting park headquarters at 540-999-3500. Bring two filled-out copies of your permit, and deposit one copy in the self-registration box at each entrance station. The other copy should be affixed to your pack or tent in full view when in the backcountry.

Backcountry Camping Regulations

1. You must have a free backcountry camping permit (see previous page).

2. Food, trash, and scented items must be stored in a tree at least 10 feet above the ground and 4 feet out from a tree trunk, within a park-approved bear-resistant food storage canister, or from a food storage pole provided at backcountry huts on the AT.

3. Backcountry campfires are not permitted.

4. A few specific areas in the park are completely closed to backcountry camping: **Old Rag Mountain** above 2,800 feet, most of **Little Stony Man Mountain, Hawksbill** above 3,600 feet, **Mary's Rock** summit, **North Mount Marshall** summit area, a portion of **Whiteoak Canyon**, and around **Overall Run Falls.** Other areas where backcountry camping is prohibited include the clearings of **Big Meadows** and within 0.5 mile of **Camp Rapidan.** If you're planning a hiking trip and/or a backcountry overnight trip to one of those areas, check the park's website for precise maps of closed areas: nps.gov/shen/planyourvisit/campbc_regs.htm.

5. Look for a legal, comfortable, and safe place to camp: one that protects the park as well as the solitude of other hikers and campers. A common strategy is to choose a preexisting campsite—that is, a site that was created and established by previous visitors and is not posted, signed, or officially designated by the park. Look for a preexisting site at least 20 yards from a trail or an unpaved fire road.

   If you can't locate a preexisting campsite, you may camp on a previously undisturbed area. Limit your stay to one night; camp well out of sight of trails, roads, and other camping groups; and practice Leave No Trace principles (see lnt.org for more information):

   • Properly dispose of human waste.

   • Limit maximum group size to 10 individuals.

   • Pack out all trash and dispose of it properly.

   Another backcountry option is a hut or cabin maintained by the **Potomac Appalachian Trail Club (PATC)** inside the park. Huts are three-sided structures located along the AT and are intended for use by hikers who are on the trail for three consecutive nights or more. Backcountry camping permits are required for camping in huts, and all Shenandoah backcountry camping regulations apply. Permits aren't required for cabins, which must be reserved in advance with the PATC (call 703-242-0315, ext. 102, or visit patc.net for more information).

   A fourth option for AT hikers is a designated campsite: a park-constructed site that provides overflow camping space near an occupied AT hut. Designated campsites are marked with a post bearing a tent symbol.

6. No camping may occur (a) within 10 yards of a stream or other natural water source; (b) within 50 yards of standing building ruins including stone foundations, chimneys, and log walls; (c) within 50 yards of another camping party or a NO CAMPING post or sign; (d) within 0.25 mile of a paved road, park boundary, or park facilities such as a campground, picnic area, visitor center, lodge, wayside, or restaurant; or (e) within 100 yards of a hut, cabin, or day-use shelter, except at designated campsites as described above.

7. Pets must be leashed at all times and are prohibited altogether on some hiking trails. Hikes where pets are not allowed are indicated throughout the book.

8. Campers may not exceed 2 consecutive nights in one location or 14 consecutive nights total in the backcountry.

Geography and Topography

The topography of Shenandoah results from the weathering of one of the oldest mountain ranges in the world—the Appalachians. Shenandoah National Park overlays a long stretch of the Blue Ridge, whose billion-year-old rocks rise above the forest. The main spine of the park stretches 70 miles from end to end, dividing the bucolic Shenandoah Valley from the Piedmont to the east. Elevations vary from 4,050 feet atop Hawksbill down to less than 550 feet near Front Royal. This vertical variation is one of the reasons for the incredible diversity of life found within its boundaries.

Shenandoah National Park forms the headwaters to many a stream flowing west and east from the north-to-south-oriented Blue Ridge. The South Fork Shenandoah River system absorbs all waterways spilling west from the park. The South Fork meets the North Fork Shenandoah River just north of the park, melding their waters and contributing them to the Potomac River, which in turn flows through the District of Columbia to the sea. The streams draining to the east are a little more complicated. Tributaries of the Rivanna River, including the Doyles and Moormans Rivers, flow from the mountains of the South District to meet the James River, which flows through Richmond to the sea. In the Central District, the Rapidan River and its tributaries from the South River to the Thornton River find their way to the Piedmont and the Rappahannock River, which flows through Fredericksburg before pushing into Chesapeake Bay. In the North District, smaller streams also course east into the headwaters of the Rappahannock and beyond.

The dominant landform is the high, continuous ridge extending north–south from one end of Shenandoah to the other: the Blue Ridge. In addition to dividing river drainages, it also forms the boundary for numerous Old Dominion counties. Often-rocky shoulder ridges, like ribs protruding from a backbone, extend from the Blue Ridge and separate steep, deeply wooded valleys carved out by eons of precipitation.

Flora

Shenandoah harbors plant species from throughout the Appalachian chain, from the hardwoods of the South to evergreens normally found in boreal climes, clinging to the highest points. Of course, the trees are the most visible piece of these complex ecosystems, gently overlapping and intermingling. Below the canopy rises more plant life. The Shenandoah you see today is the result of park protection, for much of this preserve was razed and used as pasture. There are few old-growth stands of trees; however, sporadic old-growth giants can be found along many trails. But the native ecosystems have reclaimed their rightful spots on the mountains. It's not just the showy trees and wildflowers blooming throughout the warm season that get attention; Shenandoah also displays amazing arrays of humble yet biologically important plants from mosses to fungi.

This diverse plant mosaic blends and divides depending on elevation, precipitation, and exposure. The great oak forests of Shenandoah are a starting point: growing along the ridges and slopes of the mountains, red and chestnut oaks stand sturdy while producing fall mast for wildlife. Mountain laurel, dogwood, and scraggly pines often accompany the great oaks. In the park's lower reaches grow Southern temperate woodlands, an agglomeration of hardwoods from sourwood to sassafras in drier areas. Cove hardwoods tower over lower reaches in hollows, dominated by tulip trees. Along the streams towering white pines, black birch, and mountain laurel provide shade. The hemlocks have been decimated by the hemlock woolly adelgid. Some stands and individual trees have been preserved, and we hope they will regenerate in the future.

On the higher ridges with cooler, moister conditions and the highest elevation watersheds, the vegetation morphs into northern hardwoods, such as yellow birch, beech, and cherry. Rise still higher, and you will occasionally find red spruce or Fraser fir trees, the two northern-climate trees that hug the highest peaks of the Appalachians, where it is still cool enough for them to survive. Shenandoah has no great stretches of boreal forest, just small pockets of trees sprinkled in the highlands. Throughout the park, locust, pine, and brambles continue reclaiming former clearings, transforming them into towering woodlands once again. Together these forest types, blending and intermingling, comprise a diverse biological ecosystem worthy of national park protection.

Fauna

The Shenandoah's rich flora and large wildlands support an impressive array of mammals—more than 50 species. The black bear roams throughout

Shenandoah and is commonly encountered. From the rich acorn crops of the oak forests to the fruit trees from pioneer homesteads to berries growing rampant in former fields, bears have a wide variety of food sources within the park. Don't be surprised if you come across a bruin.

There is no doubt that you will see white-tailed deer. When the park was populated by pioneers, unregulated hunting nearly drove the deer from Shenandoah, but today they are found along Skyline Drive and beyond. Drivers must constantly look out for these gentle creatures. They can also be found in the woods and especially in historically cleared areas such as Big Meadows.

A quiet hiker may also witness turkeys on wooded hillsides or in clearings. Furtive bobcats can sometimes be spotted crossing trails. Raccoons are occasionally seen in the wild. Coyotes, found throughout the park, will usually spot you before you see them. A bounding tan tail disappearing into the distance will likely comprise a sighting of this critter, which effectively replaced the extirpated red wolf in the East.

Extensive efforts have been made to keep all animals wild in Shenandoah. Long gone are the days of roadside feedings. Education, along with bearproof garbage cans and storage containers, has reduced negative interactions between people and wildlife.

More than 200 bird species either live in the park or migrate through it. These avians, including pileated woodpeckers and red-tailed hawks, ply the forest for food. The Eastern screech owl emits a goose bump–raising call. Songbirds native to the north and south find a home in the park, and Shenandoah's north–south orientation adds to its importance as a migratory-bird corridor. Birding, a popular pastime in the park, can enhance any hike.

The park's waters harbor about three dozen types of fish. Most famously, Shenandoah is a bastion for brook trout. Unlike the Smokies, this park has never had rainbow or brook trout intentionally introduced into its waters.

Rattlesnakes *may be encountered on the trail—especially in sunny, rocky areas.*

"Brookies" are the only trout native to Shenandoah. Technically, the brook is not a true trout, but a char. Brooks prefer cold, clear waters and are found in more than 50 of the park's 90 streams. Brown trout have been making their way into the lower reaches of Shenandoah's streams, but biologists are trying to limit their numbers.

Spend some time hiking at Shenandoah, and you may be surprised by the variety of snakes in the area: 18 species in all. Most of those you encounter will be non-venomous, but be aware that two kinds of poisonous snakes—the copperhead and the timber rattler—call the park home. Copperheads can be found near streams and on outcrops, whereas rattlers will primarily be seen sunning on rocks.

Shenandoah also harbors 14 types of salamanders, including the rare Shenandoah salamander, found only within the park. It's just one more example of how the life in these mountains lives up to its national park status.

When to Go

Shenandoah has a somewhat undeserved reputation of being overcrowded. Yes, Skyline Drive and its overlooks and facilities can be crowded during summer, on warm season weekends, and on holidays. And it's true that the roads can also be busy during the October leaf-viewing season. Get a quarter mile from a trailhead on 95% of the hiking trails, however, and you'll experience solitude. Busy trails—and there are a number of them—are noted in the trail descriptions.

Shenandoah National Park is a four-season destination. Hikers with well-thought-out plans can easily execute their treks beyond the obvious busy times. Try to hike midweek and just before or after major holidays. Spring is a great time, with its renewing vibrancy exemplified by colorful wildflowers and budding trees, as the season of renewal climbs the mountains from low to high. Fall can be rewarding, too, but avoid October weekends. Solitude can be found anytime during winter. As far as busy trails go, try to hike them early in the morning or later in the evening. Iffy weather—that is, a 50% or more chance of rain—often keeps the crowds away. If you can, avoid busy trails on nice-weather weekends.

Weather and Seasons

Each of the four distinct seasons lays its hands on Shenandoah National Park, though elevation always factors into park weather patterns. While each season brings exciting changes in the flora and fauna, the changes can occur seemingly day to day rather than month to month.

Be prepared for a wide range of temperatures and conditions regardless of the season. As a rule of thumb, the temperature decreases about 3 degrees for every 1,000 feet of elevation gained. The approximately 50 inches of yearly precipitation on the Blue Ridge is about 15 inches more than the nearby Shenandoah Valley receives. This precipitation is evenly distributed throughout the year, though it arrives with slow-moving frontal systems in winter and with thunderstorms in summer.

The table below lists temperatures at Luray, Virginia, in the Shenandoah Valley just west of the park. Expect temperatures in the higher park elevations to be 10 degrees cooler.

Average High and Low Temperature by Month: Luray, Virginia						
	JAN	FEB	MARCH	APRIL	MAY	JUNE
High	46°F	50°F	59°F	71°F	78°F	85°F
Low	23°F	25°F	31°F	39°F	48°F	56°F
	JULY	AUG	SEPT	OCT	NOV	DEC
High	88°F	86°F	81°F	71°F	61°F	50°F
Low	60°F	59°F	52°F	41°F	34°F	25°F

Spring is the most variable season. During March, the first signs of rebirth appear in the lowlands, yet trees in the high country may not fully leaf out until June. Visitors can experience both winter- and summerlike weather in spring. As summer approaches, the strong fronts weaken, and thunderstorms and haze become more frequent. Summertime rainy days can be cool. In fall, continental fronts once again sweep through, clearing the air and bringing warm days and cool nights, though rain is always possible.

The first snows of winter usually arrive in November, and snow can intermittently fall through April, though no permanent snowpack exists. About 40–120 inches of snow can fall during this time. Expect to incur entire days of below-freezing weather, though temperatures can range from mild to bitterly cold, often depending on the elevation.

About the Trails

Trail Selection

Four criteria were used to select the trails for this guide. Only the premier day hikes and overnight backpacks are included, based upon the most beautiful scenery, unique Shenandoah features, ease of access, and diversity of experience. Some of the selected trails are very popular; others are used more infrequently.

Key Features

Top Trails books contain information about features for each trail, such as old-growth trees, waterfalls, great views, and more. Shenandoah National Park is blessed with an incredible diversity of terrain and associated flora and fauna—no matter what your interests, you're sure to find a trail to match them. Hikes range throughout the vast variety of ecosystems, from the spruce–fir pockets to the great oak forests to the deep canyons where verdant streams house waterfalls tumbling still deeper into the back of beyond. Those who love a view will find plenty of rock outcrops, meadows, and other vista points where rewarding views can be had. Photographers will be glad that we live in the age of the digital camera and handy smartphone, since they can shoot limitless pictures of showy spring wildflowers and vibrant fall-color panoramas.

Campgrounds, cabins, and lodges throughout the park make for great base camps for hikers. Backcountry camping allows hikers to extend their trips beyond day hiking. Anglers can toss a line in more than 50 fishable waterways. Some Shenandoah streams also harbor swimming holes. Wildlife can be seen in the clearings of Big Meadows and other places between.

Multiple Uses

All of the trails described in this guide are suitable for hiking. Some of the trails can also be enjoyed by equestrians, though the number of horseback enthusiasts in Shenandoah is far outstripped by hikers. Very few trails see more than sporadic equestrian use, though the Skyland area offers guided rides during the warm season. Bicyclists are relegated to Skyline Drive and paved roads, except for a mile-long stretch of Rapidan Fire Road. Fishing is done primarily along backcountry streams.

Unlike most national parks, Shenandoah allows pets on the vast majority of its backcountry trails, provided they're on a 6-foot leash. Certain paths that don't allow pets are signed as such and are noted in the trails tables and elsewhere in the book.

On the Trail

E very outing should begin with proper preparation, which usually takes only a few minutes. Even the easiest trail can turn up unexpected surprises. People seldom think about getting lost or injured, but unexpected things can and do happen. Simple precautions can make the difference between a good story and a dangerous situation.

Have a Plan

Before You Go

Choose Wisely The first step to enjoying any trail is to match the trail to your abilities. It's no use overestimating your experience or fitness—know your abilities and limitations, and use the Top Trails difficulty rating that accompanies each trail.

Leave Word About Your Plans The most basic of precautions is leaving word of your intentions with friends or family. Many people will hike the backcountry their entire lives without ever relying on this safety net, but establishing this simple habit is free insurance.

It's best to leave specific information—location, trail name, intended time of travel—with a responsible person. It takes but a minute to shoot a friend or loved one a text. If, however, this isn't possible or if your plans change at the last minute, you should still leave word. If there's a ranger station, trail register, or visitor center, check in.

Review the Route Before embarking on any hike, *read the entire description and study the map*. It isn't necessary to memorize every detail, but you do want to have a clear mental picture of the trail and general area.

 Prepare and Plan

- Know your abilities and limitations.
- Leave word about your plans.
- Know your route and the area.

Because virtually all of the described trails are well used and easy to follow, a supplemental topographic map isn't a must, but for those who prefer to use them, a list of U.S. Geological Survey topos is provided at the beginning of each chapter.

Carry the Essentials

Proper preparation for any type of trail use also includes gathering certain essential items to carry. Your trip checklist will vary according to trail choice and conditions.

Clothing When the weather is good, light, comfortable clothing is the obvious choice. It's easy to believe that very little spare clothing is needed, but a prepared hiker has something tucked away for any emergency from a surprise shower to an unexpected overnight in a remote area.

Clothing includes proper footwear, essential for hiking and running trails. As a trail becomes more demanding, you will need footwear that performs. Running shoes are fine for many trails. If you will be carrying substantial weight or encountering sustained rugged terrain, step up to hiking boots.

Shenandoah can be notoriously humid in summer. Hikers often sweat more than normal. Breathable, moisture-wicking clothes will help keep you cool and dry. In cooler weather, particularly when it's wet, carry waterproof outer garments and quick-drying undergarments (avoid cotton). Shenandoah can also be a rainy place. Unless the forecast calls for absolutely no chance of rain, bring a rain jacket or poncho. As general rule, whatever the conditions, bring layers that can be combined or removed to provide comfort and protection from the elements in a wide variety of conditions.

Water Never embark on a trail without carrying water. At all times, particularly in warm weather, adequate water is of key importance. Experts recommend at least 2 quarts of water per day; when hiking in heat, a gallon or more may be more appropriate. At the extreme, dehydration can be life-threatening. More commonly, inadequate water brings fatigue and muscle aches.

For most outings, unless the day is very hot or the trail very long, you should plan to carry sufficient water for the entire trail. Unfortunately, in North America natural water sources are questionable, and generally loaded with various risks: bacteria, viruses, and fertilizers.

Trail Essentials

- Dress to keep cool, but be ready for cold.
- Carry plenty of water.
- Have adequate food (plus a little extra).

Water Treatment If you find yourself needing to make use of trailside water, you'll want to treat it before you drink it. There are three treatment methods: boiling, chemicals, and filtering. Boiling is the most effective but often impractical—it requires a heat source, a pot, and plenty of time. Chemical treatments, available at outdoors stores, take care of some problems, including the troublesome giardia parasite, but they won't combat many artificial chemical pollutants, plus they tend to add an unpleasant aftertaste. The preferred method is filtration, which removes giardia and other contaminants minus the chemical aftertaste. Today's filters, such as those made by Sawyer, are small, lightweight, and inexpensive.

If this hasn't convinced you to carry all the water you need, here's one final admonishment: be prepared for surprises. Water sources described in the text or shown on maps can change course or dry up completely. Never let your water bottle run dry in expectation of the next source—fill up wherever water is available, and always keep a little in reserve.

Food While not as critical as water, food is energy and its importance shouldn't be underestimated. Avoid foods that are hard to digest, such as candy bars and potato chips. Carry high energy, fast-digesting foods: nutrition bars, dehydrated fruit, trail mix, and jerky. Bring a little more food that you think you'll need—it's good to bring along on an outing that turns unexpectedly long, perhaps because of inclement weather or losing your way.

Useful but Less-Than-Essential Items

Map and Compass (and the Know-How to Use Them) Many trails don't require much navigation, meaning that a map and compass aren't always as essential as water or food—but it can be a close judgment call. If the trail is remote or infrequently visited, a map and compass should be considered necessities.

A dedicated GPS receiver is also a useful trail companion. While it's no substitute for a map and compass, a GPS, along with downloaded topographic maps, is good to have in your navigational toolbox. The drawback is batteries dying or the device otherwise becoming unusable.

Smartphone Much of the Blue Ridge and lowlands near towns and along the roads that cross Shenandoah have some level of cellular coverage. In many areas, however, especially in hollows and along streams, there is no service at all. In extreme circumstances, a smartphone can be a lifesaver as a GPS unit and communication device, but you shouldn't depend on it—coverage is unpredictable, especially deep in the hollows. As with a dedicated GPS, smartphone batteries run out of juice eventually, so before you make a call or fire up your mapping app, make sure it's warranted—a blister doesn't justify a call to search-and-rescue.

Gear Depending on the remoteness and rigor of the trail, there are many additional useful items to consider: pocketknife, flashlight, fire source (waterproof matches, light, or flint), and a first aid kit. Every member of your party should carry the appropriate essential items described above; groups often split up or get separated along the trail. Solo hikers should be even more disciplined about preparation and carry more gear. Traveling solo is inherently more risky. This isn't meant to discourage solo travel, but rather to emphasize the need for extra preparation.

Trail Etiquette

The overriding rule on the trail is **Leave No Trace.** This is especially applicable to the more popular hiking destinations in and about Shenandoah National Park, where certain waterfalls and overlooks will be visited by hundreds of hikers.

Never Litter If you carried it in, it's even easier to carry it out, since it weighs less. Try picking up any litter you encounter and packing it out—it's a rewarding feeling. Nature also litters, and I make it a habit to move at least a bit of debris from the trail, be it boulders, branches, or small trees. It is amazing just how large a tree a few sturdy hikers can move.

Don't Build Campsites Constructing your own camp furniture or clearing the ground to place a tent or tarp transforms a pristine site into a human one— hardly a wilderness experience. Also, if you're going cross-country, don't mark your route. Let others do their own rewarding pathfinding just as you did.

Stay on the Trail Repeated shortcutting of switchbacks can lead to rapid erosion and time-consuming trail repair, costing taxpayer dollars. Also, because shortcuts are steeper and have an uneven, sometimes bouldery tread, they can be dangerous, particularly for an exhausted backpacker in a hurry to get down. Don't risk broken bones or sprained ankles.

Share the Trail Shenandoah's trails attract many visitors, so be prepared to share the trail with them. Commonly accepted trail etiquette dictates that

---

Trail Etiquette

- Leave no trace—Never litter.
- Stay on the trail—Never cut switchbacks.
- Share the trail—Use courtesy and common sense.
- Leave it there—Don't disturb plants or wildlife.

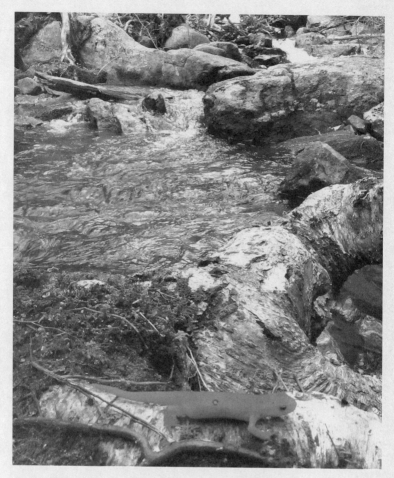

Salamander in repose *on the Hazel River (see Trail 15, page 117)*

hikers yield to equestrians and their stock, and that ascending and descending hikers keep to their respective right side as they pass each other.* Short tourist trails
host hundreds to thousands of visitors a day. You may meet an obnoxious
person or two, but don't become that person and spoil someone else's day.

Leave It There Removing or destroying plants, animals, and historical artifacts is both unethical and illegal.

CHAPTER 1

North District

North District

The North District encompasses the most northerly of Shenandoah's three ranger districts that divide the park. This section stretches from Front Royal, the northernmost boundary of Shenandoah, to Thornton Gap in the south, where US 211 bisects the park east–west while connecting Luray to Sperryville. Traveling south from Front Royal, the Blue Ridge rises with proverbial Skyline Drive winding atop it. Dickey Ridge Visitor Center is often a hiker's first stop. A popular walk starts here. South of Dickey Ridge, notable heights (Compton Peak among others) begin rising where you can see the Blue Ridge rising from adjacent lowlands.

The park widens near Mount Marshall, and then you reach Mathews Arm Campground. Here, several streams and ridges spill off both sides of the Blue Ridge, creating a large wildland. On the west side of the Blue Ridge you find Overall Run Falls—the park's highest at 93 feet—tumbling over a ragged cliff. Remote Knob Mountain and Neighbor Mountain border ultrascenic Jeremys Run, with its big pools, waterfalls, swimming holes, and everywhere-you-look beauty. The Big Devils Stairs and Little Devils Stairs are boulder-covered, rugged gorges passable only by hikers. The Piney River cuts a secluded swath between Pignut Mountain and Piney Ridge, while the North Fork Thornton River Valley recalls pioneer history with its numerous homesites. Area streams have mostly trout, but some smallmouth bass. Sycamore, white pines, and mountain laurel, along with alder thickets, border the waterways. Shenandoah's famous oak stands rise on drier ridges. Elevations range from 550 feet near Front Royal to almost 3,400 feet atop Mount Marshall in this, the smallest of the park's three districts.

The Appalachian Trail (AT) acts a spinal pathway for the North District, connecting all major watersheds, the mountains that divide them, and the trails that course through points high and low. The AT is useful for planning loop hikes in the North District. Most hikes here are accessed from Skyline Drive.

Opposite and overleaf: *Vista from outcrop near Overall Run Falls (Trail 5, page 49)*

Visitors have one overnight option in the North District—Mathews Arm Campground. You can camp here on a first-come, first-served basis, but reservations are available on one loop. The higher elevation keeps it a good 10 degrees cooler than the Shenandoah Valley below. Make sure to store your food carefully, as Mathews Arm is bear country. More civilized accommodations can be had in nearby Front Royal or Luray.

The hikes described are either loops or out-and-back treks. Along the way you can see local highlights—Little Devils Stairs, Piney River Falls, and the old farms on Dickey Ridge. Other treks travel lesser-trod trails, such as Sugarloaf and Beecher Ridge, where park beauty is more subtle.

Permits

Permits are not required for day hiking. Backpackers must get a permit to stay in the backcountry. Simple self-registration stations are located at the Front Royal Entrance Station, the Dickey Ridge Visitor Center, the north boundary where the AT leaves the park, the Panorama, and the Thornton Gap Entrance Station.

Turk's cap lily *graces the late-summer forest on the Big Devils Stairs Trail* (*Trail 3, page 39*).

North District

North District

TRAIL	Difficulty	Length	Type	USES & ACCESS	TERRAIN	NATURE	OTHER
1	2	4.3	Loop	Day Hiking, Pets Prohibited	Summit	Autumn Colors	Great Views, Historical Interest
2	3	3.2	Out-and-Back	Day Hiking	Summit, Ridgeline	Autumn Colors	Great Views, Geological Interest
3	3	5.0	Out-and-Back	Day Hiking, Backpacking	Ridgeline, Stream	Autumn Colors, Wildflowers	Great Views
4	3	4.7	Loop	Day Hiking, Backpacking	Ridgeline, Stream	Autumn Colors, Wildlife	Great Views, Geological Interest
5	4	6.8	Out-and-Back	Day Hiking	Ridgeline, Stream, Waterfall	Autumn Colors, Wildflowers, Wildlife	Great Views, Camping, Geological Interest
6	4	5.4	Loop	Day Hiking, Backpacking	Ridgeline, Stream	Autumn Colors, Wildflowers	Great Views, Historical Interest, Geological Interest
7	5	9.2	Loop	Day Hiking, Backpacking	Ridgeline, Stream, Waterfall	Autumn Colors, Wildlife	Great Views, Camping, Swimming, Secluded, Steep, Historical Interest, Geological Interest
8	4	7.2	Loop	Day Hiking, Backpacking	Ridgeline, Stream	Autumn Colors, Wildflowers, Wildlife	Camping, Secluded, Historical Interest
9	3	5.6	Loop	Day Hiking	Ridgeline, Stream	Autumn Colors, Wildflowers, Wildlife	Camping, Secluded
10	4	6.8	Out-and-Back	Day Hiking, Backpacking	Ridgeline, Stream, Waterfall	Autumn Colors, Wildflowers	Secluded
11	5	13.1	Loop	Day Hiking, Backpacking	Summit, Ridgeline, Stream, Waterfall	Autumn Colors, Wildlife	Great Views, Swimming, Secluded, Steep, Geological Interest
12	5	14.0	Loop	Day Hiking, Backpacking	Summit, Ridgeline, Stream, Waterfall	Autumn Colors, Wildflowers	Great Views, Swimming, Secluded, Steep
13	4	7.9	Loop	Day Hiking, Backpacking	Summit, Ridgeline, Stream, Waterfall	Autumn Colors, Wildflowers, Wildlife	Steep, Historical Interest

Legend

TYPE
- Loop
- Out-and-Back

DIFFICULTY
- 1 2 3 4 5 +
- less   more

USES & ACCESS
- Day Hiking
- Backpacking
- Child-Friendly
- Pets Prohibited

TERRAIN
- Summit
- Ridgeline
- Stream
- Waterfall

NATURE
- Autumn Colors
- Wildflowers
- Wildlife
- Old-Growth Forest

FEATURES
- Great Views
- Camping
- Swimming
- Secluded
- Steep
- Historical Interest
- Geological Interest

Maps

For the North District, here are the relevant U.S. Geological Survey 7.5-minute (1:24,000-scale) topographic quadrangles, listed in geographic order as you hike along your route:

Trail 1: *Chester Gap* and *Front Royal*
Trail 2: *Chester Gap*
Trail 3: *Chester Gap*
Trail 4: *Bentonville* and *Thornton Gap*
Trail 5: *Bentonville*
Trail 6: *Thornton Gap* and *Bentonville*
Trail 7: *Bentonville*
Trail 8: *Bentonville*
Trail 9: *Bentonville* and *Thornton Gap*
Trail 10: *Thornton Gap*
Trail 11: *Thornton Gap* and *Bentonville*
Trail 12: *Thornton Gap*
Trail 13: *Thornton Gap*

North District

Dickey Ridge Historic Hike. 29

Easy access, old farmsteads, and a good view sum up much of what Shenandoah National Park offers in one hike. Leave Dickey Ridge Visitor Center, and slip down to the old Fox Farm. Discover pioneer vestiges there, including a cemetery. Walk south on Dickey Ridge to Snead Farm site, and check out more human history. Catch a great view of the Shenandoah Valley on your way back, then enjoy more attractive ridgeline woodland.

TRAIL 1

Day Hiking,
Pets Prohibited
4.3 miles, Loop
Difficulty: 1 **2** 3 4 5

Compton Peak. 35

This hike takes a lesser-used approach to a mountaintop with two rewarding vistas from rock protrusions along its flanks. The Appalachian Trail climbs moderately to these panoramas. Along the way explore nature's recovery and fire ecology, where the Smith Run Fire enveloped 1,710 acres of the park.

TRAIL 2

Day Hiking
3.2 miles, Out-and-back
Difficulty: 1 2 **3** 4 5

Big Devils Stairs Vista. 39

This moderate hike leads to a great reward, with plenty of solitude along the way. The nearly level Bluff Trail leads to the Big Devils Stairs canyon rim for a deep view of the valley below and the mountains beyond. At the hike's outset, pass a shelter used by long-distance hikers on the Appalachian Trail.

TRAIL 3

Day Hiking,
Backpacking
5.0 miles, Out-and-back
Difficulty: 1 2 **3** 4 5

Heiskell Hollow Loop 67

This Mathews Arm area trek has no single superlative feature to draw in hikers but offers solitude aplenty. Hike secluded Beecher Ridge, traveling the spine of this regally forested highland before picking up the Heiskell Hollow Trail. Plenty of pioneer evidence awaits a sharp-eyed hiker.

TRAIL 8

Day Hiking,
Backpacking
7.2 miles, Loop
Difficulty: 1 2 3 **4** 5

Elkwallow Loop 71

This classic Shenandoah circuit first navigates a boulder field before making a pleasantly level highland track on the Blue Ridge. Eventually dip to Jeremys Run. Pick up the seldom-trod Knob Mountain Trail on a remarkably level track to finish the circuit.

TRAIL 9

Day Hiking
5.6 miles, Loop
Difficulty: 1 2 **3** 4 5

Piney River Falls 75

The scenery on this solitude-laden hike meets high Shenandoah standards, and the falls are a worthy destination. Gently wind your way through eye-pleasing, high-country woods to the Piney River Valley and the three-tier falls.

TRAIL 10

Day Hiking,
Backpacking
6.8 miles, Out-and-back
Difficulty: 1 2 3 **4** 5

Knob Mountain and Jeremys Run Loop 81

This is a long yet rewarding loop exploring points high and low. Traverse Knob Mountain, soaking in views en route to Jeremys Run. Make your way up gorgeous Jeremys Run valley, crossing the stream more than a dozen times. Don't expect company on Knob Mountain, though you may see a few people along Jeremys Run.

TRAIL 11

Day Hiking,
Backpacking
13.1 miles, Loop
Difficulty: 1 2 3 4 **5**

Even turtles *love the trails of Shenandoah.*

Dickey Ridge Historic Hike

Easy access, old farmsteads, and a good view piece together a nice family or group hike that sums up much of what Shenandoah National Park offers. Leave the Dickey Ridge Visitor Center, and slip down to the old Fox Farm, which has many pioneer vestiges, including a cemetery. Walk south on Dickey Ridge. Walk south to the Snead Farm site, and check out more human history. Make a rewarding woodland walk. Catch a great view of the Shenandoah Valley on your way back, then enjoy more attractive hilltop woodland. *Note:* Pets are *not* allowed on this trail.

Best Time

After the leaves fall—winter through early spring—is the best time for this hike. This is when you can best see the ample evidence of pre-park residents. Summer can be warm and busy.

Finding the Trail

The hike starts at the Dickey Ridge Visitor Center, milepost 4.6 on Skyline Drive. From the Front Royal Entrance Station, head south on Skyline Drive 4.6 miles to the visitor center.

Trail Description

Leave the visitor center near the flagpole. ▶1 Interestingly, the visitor center was originally a dining hall for a set of now-demolished rental cabins, built in the early days of Shenandoah National Park.

TRAIL USE
Day Hiking,
Pets Prohibited
LENGTH
4.3 miles, 2.5–3.5 hours
VERTICAL FEET
±700'
DIFFICULTY
– 1 **2** 3 4 5 +
TRAIL TYPE
Loop
START & FINISH
N38° 52.296'
W78° 12.273'

FEATURES
Ridgeline
Autumn Colors
Great Views
Historical Interest

FACILITIES
Picnic tables
Restrooms
Visitor center
Water

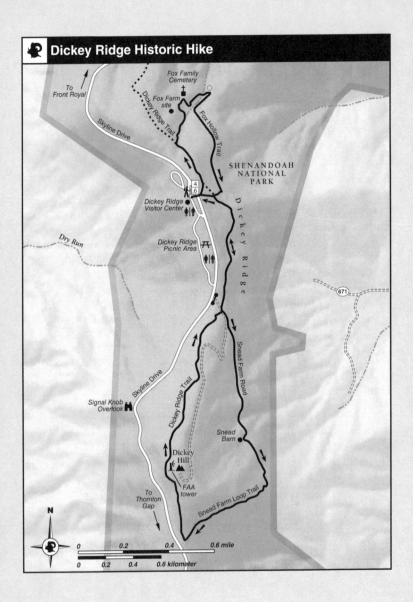

Dickey Ridge Historic Hike

To Front Royal

Fox Family Cemetery

Fox Farm site

Dickey Ridge Trail

Fox Hollow Trail

SHENANDOAH NATIONAL PARK

Skyline Drive

4 6

Dickey Ridge Visitor Center

D i c k e y   R i d g e

Dry Run

Dickey Ridge Picnic Area

671

Skyline Drive

Snead Farm Road

Signal Knob Overlook

Dickey Ridge Trail

Snead Barn

Dickey Hill

FAA tower

Snead Farm Loop Trail

To Thornton Gap

N

| 0 | 0.2 | 0.4 | 0.6 mile |

| 0 | 0.2 | 0.4 | 0.6 kilometer |

OPTION

For a short historical stroll, walk the Dickey Ridge and Fox Hollow Loop, returning to the Dickey Ridge Visitor Center after 1.3 miles, with an elevation change of only 250 feet.

Cross Skyline Drive. Easterly views open beyond the grassy hill in front of you. You can purchase an interpretive pamphlet here. Turn left at an informational sign, walk a short distance, and then join the Dickey Ridge Trail, entering woodland. The hardwood forest here is covered in vines. At 0.3 mile, turn right on the Fox Hollow Trail. ▶2 As you descend into Fox Hollow, you see walls of rock, relics of the farms that were here before the brushy woods came to occupy the site. Look at the large stone edifice, placed there by generations of Foxes toiling the terrain, clearing the land to increase fertility and yield. More rock walls stand down the trail.

At 0.5 mile, come to the Fox family cemetery. ▶3 Bordered by fieldstones and cloaked in periwinkle, the graveyard is a somber reminder that this land was many things to many people before it became a national park. (The name Dickey Ridge, in fact, appears in records dating back to before the United States was established.) Soon pass a spring enclosed in concrete. This spring, once used by Foxes, was encased in concrete only after the national park drew water for the dining hall–turned–visitor center. Ahead, embedded in the ground, lies a decorative millstone, once made to grind corn elsewhere, but used as a decorative step by the Foxes. The trail bisects the spring outflow and then switches back, passing a rusty wire fence.

It then picks up an old road connecting Dickey Ridge to Front Royal at 0.7 mile. The loop turns south and scrambles uphill in brushy woods before

 Historical Interest

Explore Shenandoah's past on this great family hike.

rejoining the Dickey Ridge Trail at 1.3 miles. ▶4 The visitor center stands just above you.

To continue the longer double loop, stay with the gentle Dickey Ridge Trail. It cruises through more vine-covered woods. Watch for a rock fence that runs along a steep slope left of the trail. There weren't many out-of-shape farmers in these Potomac Highlands. At 1.9 miles, reach the junction with Snead Farm Road. Turn left here, joining a blue-blazed gravel track. ▶5 Then come to three signed road forks. At the first fork, take the road to the left—the road right leads to a Federal Aviation Administration (FAA) flight-tracking station. At the second fork, take the road to the right—the left fork goes to the water station for Dickey Ridge Visitor Center and its picnic area. Just ahead, look for an old bricked-in spring to the right of the roadbed. At the third fork, take the road to the left. Stay under a transmission line.

At 2.4 miles, come to a clearing with the white Snead Barn and the concrete-and-stone foundation of a house. ▶6 Ol' Snead was a relative newcomer to what became the park. The former judge owned the place only a few years before the park bought him out. The function of the cellar behind the barn has been lost to time. Explore to find the spring.

At the edge of the clearing, turn left on the Snead Farm Loop Trail. This path runs level a short

Ridgeline ▲

Dickey Ridge Historic Hike Elevation Profile

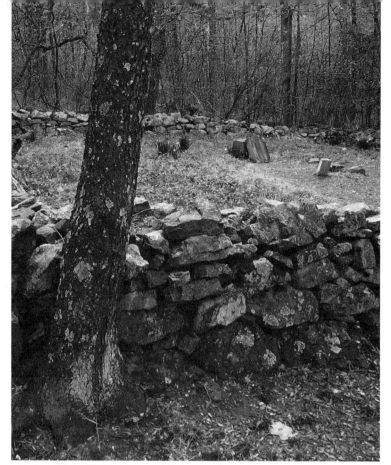

Primitive stone walls *border the cemetery at Fox Farm.*

distance and then makes an irregular climb in rocky hardwoods before meeting the Dickey Ridge Trail at 3.2 miles. ▶7 Turn right on the Dickey Ridge Trail, topping out in 0.3 mile. Stay left here as a trail leads right to the top of a knob and the aforementioned FAA airplane-tracking station. The trail descends. At 3.6 miles, come to a cleared overlook of the Shenandoah Valley, South Fork Shenandoah River, and Massanutten Mountain. ▶8

The trail rises briefly once again before making a prolonged descent through a very pleasant forest of oak, hickory, maple, basswood, and other trees. Reach Snead Farm Road and the Dickey Ridge Trail

Autumn Colors

Great Views

at 4.3 miles. ▶9 From here, it's about a half-mile meander back through the grass and trees of the Dickey Ridge Picnic Ground. This mileage is not included in the overall hike, as there are multiple routes through the picnic ground.

🚶 MILESTONES

▶ 1   0.0   Dickey Ridge Visitor Center at milepost 4.6
▶ 2   0.3   Right on Fox Hollow Trail
▶ 3   0.5   Fox Cemetery
▶ 4   1.3   Complete Fox Hollow Loop, and go straight on Dickey Ridge Trail
▶ 5   1.9   Left on Snead Farm Road
▶ 6   2.4   Snead Barn and homesite
▶ 7   3.2   Right on Dickey Ridge Trail
▶ 8   3.6   Vista
▶ 9   4.3   Reach Snead Farm Road and Dickey Ridge Trail at south end of picnic area. Meander back to visitor center.

Compton Peak

This out-and-back day hike takes the lesser-used approach to a mountaintop, with two good vistas from rock protrusions along its flanks. The Appalachian Trail (AT) is your host along the way to these two outcrops.

Best Time

For this highland vista hike, the clearer the sky, the better the views.

Finding the Trail

From Front Royal, take Skyline Drive south 12.4 miles to the Jenkins Gap Parking Area, located on the right at milepost 12.4 on Skyline Drive, just before the Jenkins Gap Overlook, which is on the left (east). The hike starts on the Jenkins Gap Trail, which leaves from the parking area, not the overlook.

Trail Description

Begin this walk on the Jenkins Gap Trail. ▶1 The yellow-blazed pathway leaves from the parking area around auto-sized boulders to intersect the AT in 164 feet. Turn right, heading northbound. The walking is easy in a mixed forest of sassafras, pin cherry, locust, and ever-present oak, shading a brushy forest floor. The signs of a 2011 fire are becoming harder to spot, though brushy, even aged trees are an indicator. Plenty of tall trees survived the burn. Keep a level track through Jenkins Gap. Enjoy the easy cruise. Skyline Drive lies to your

TRAIL USE
Day Hiking
LENGTH
3.2 miles, 2–3 hours
VERTICAL FEET
±560'
DIFFICULTY
– 1 2 **3** 4 5 +
TRAIL TYPE
Out-and-back
START & FINISH
N38° 48.395'
W78° 10.854'

FEATURES
Summit
Ridgeline
Autumn Colors
Great Views
Geological Interest

FACILITIES
None

Autumn Colors

Compton Peak

SHENANDOAH
NATIONAL
PARK

To
Front Royal

Skyline Drive

Indian Run
Overlook

Compton
Peak

Skyline Drive

Jenkins Gap Trail

P

12
4

Jenkins Gap
Overlook

Skyline Drive

To
Thornton Gap

N

0   0.1   0.2   0.3 mile

0   0.1 0.2   0.3 kilometer

right. After a while you may begin to wonder about the climb to Compton Peak. Finally, after 0.5 mile, the trail veers left and ascends a mountainside of chestnut oak and mountain laurel. ▶2

Swing around the southwest side of Compton Peak. Switchback on some elaborate stone steps built during a trail reroute. The trail regains the ridgecrest. Southward views of North Mount Marshall and South Mount Marshall open. Step over a little spring branch at 0.9 mile. ▶3 Look for apple trees persisting in the forest beyond the spring. These are remnants of an orchard on the north and south side of Jenkins Gap. I have seen a bear harvesting apples while hiking here during late summer. The AT curves past the head of the spring, angling higher.

Pass through a flat then climb a bit more to reach a four-way trail junction at 1.3 miles. ▶4 Both left and right lead to vistas. Head left on the blue-blazed trail, to the more popular and widespread view. Briefly continue climbing a stony track over a rock knob before dipping to an outcrop with a widespread vista at 1.5 miles. ▶5 Below, the track of Skyline Drive, including Gooney Run Overlook, is evident as it snakes downhill along Dickey Ridge. To the far left are the South Fork of the Shenandoah River and the

 Ridgeline

This climb to
a first-rate vista
isn't too steep.

 Summit

 Great Views

Compton Peak Elevation Profile

Shenandoah Valley. Ahead, more mountains and the flatlands extend toward Washington, DC. This is a truly inspiring vista.

The second vista is more challenging to reach and less inspiring. If you have made it this far, go ahead and check out the second view. Backtrack to reach the AT and keep forward, now on the second blue-blazed path. The trail is fainter as it goes down, down, down on a rocky tread. Reach an outcrop where you might expect a vista, but keep hiking. Hike down the bluff, walk a few feet through the woods, and scramble up a rocky prominence at mile 1.9. ►6 This prominence, an example of columnar jointing, offers worthy views of Mount Marshall in the foreground and lands east

Great Views 👀

of the Blue Ridge. While thinking of the unfortunate people who skip this second view, as evidenced by its less-used trail, the return trip to the AT will get you huffing and puffing. The blue-blazed trail now leads to the base of this prominence and then dead-ends. From this overlook, it's a simple backtrack to the trailhead. ►7

🚶	MILESTONES	
► 1	0.0	Jenkins Gap Trail Parking Area at milepost 12.4
► 2	0.5	Ascend from Jenkins Gap
► 3	0.9	Spring
► 4	1.3	Four-way split to vistas
► 5	1.5	Northwest vista
► 6	1.9	Southeast vista
► 7	3.2	Jenkins Gap Trail Parking Area at milepost 12.4

Big Devils Stairs Vista

This unsung and mostly easy hike delivers a great reward. The walking is easy, and the trails are used surprisingly little. The nearly level Bluff Trail leads to the Big Devils Stairs canyon rim for a great view of the valley below and the mountains beyond. At the hike's outset, you will pass a shelter used by long-distance hikers on the Appalachian Trail (AT).

Best Time

Even though this hike culminates in a view, it is primarily of a canyon, rather than distant mountains and valleys. Therefore, it is good any time of year.

Finding the Trail

The Gravel Springs Gap Parking Area is at milepost 17.6 on the east side of Skyline Drive. The yellow-blazed access road to Gravel Springs Hut leaves the rear of the parking area.

Trail Description

A large trailhead signboard shows the web of paths in the immediate area. Leave Skyline Drive from the rear of the Gravel Springs Gap Parking Area on the gated access road leading down to Gravel Springs Hut. ▶1 The AT leaves from the parking area as well. The southbound portion of the AT roughly parallels the access road, while the northbound AT crosses Skyline Drive here at Gravel Springs Gap. The walking is easy on the fire road, bordered by locust, apple trees, and ample brush. You are working downhill.

TRAIL USE
Day Hiking,
Backpacking

LENGTH
5.0 miles, 3–4 hours

VERTICAL FEET
±690'

DIFFICULTY
– 1 2 **3** 4 5 +

TRAIL TYPE
Out-and-back

START & FINISH
N38° 46.085'
W78° 14.000'

FEATURES
Ridgeline
Stream
Autumn Colors
Wildflowers
Great Views

FACILITIES
None

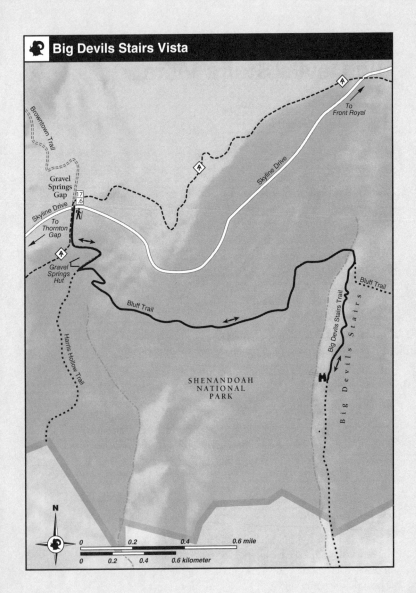

Big Devils Stairs Vista

Browntown Trail

Gravel
Springs
Gap

17.6

Skyline Drive

To
Thornton
Gap

Gravel
Springs
Hut

Bluff Trail

Harris Hollow Trail

SHENANDOAH
NATIONAL
PARK

Skyline Drive

To
Front Royal

Bluff Trail

Big Devils Stairs Trail

Big Devils Stairs

N

0   0.2   0.4   0.6 mile

0   0.2   0.4   0.6 kilometer

After a quarter mile, the trail makes a switch-back to the left and the Harris Hollow Trail leads left to the Bluff Trail, your destination. The horse trail allows equestrian access to the Bluff Trail without going to Gravel Springs Hut. Stay right with the roadbed, drifting down to Gravel Springs at 0.4 mile. ►2 You will see the rocked-in upwelling to your right. The three-sided trail shelter, fronted by a fireplace, stands just beyond. Primarily of stone and wood construction, these trail shelters are based roughly 10 miles apart the entire length of the AT, including here at Shenandoah National Park. Imagine staying in shelters like this one on the 2,100-mile trek from Georgia to Maine.

This hike continues on the Bluff Trail, which leaves the shelter clearing near Gravel Springs. Pass the Harris Hollow Trail coming from Gravel Springs Gap. Make a big switchback ahead, step-ping over a spring branch. At 0.6 mile, the Harris Hollow Trail leaves right. Again, the Harris Hollow Trail is working around Gravel Springs and the trail shelter so that horses won't foul the spring. Stay with the Bluff Trail, recrossing the spring branch. From here, it runs nearly level, around 2,300 feet, on the southeast slope of Mount Marshall beneath a high-canopied forest of multitrunked basswood, oak, and hickory strewn with large boulders, low bluffs, and outcrops.

Wildflowers

At 1.1 miles, the forest opens on the right amid rock, offering views to the south. Ahead, several branches cross the trail and meet the main stem flowing from Gravel Springs. They all ultimately flow into the Rush River, outside the park. Many of these will be dry in late summer and fall. At 1.8 miles, step over the upper reaches of the stream that runs through Big Devils Stairs Gorge, which is just beginning to cut its way down the mountainside. ►3 This unnamed tributary, also a branch of the Rush River, is an easy crossing in times of normal water

Big Devils Stairs canyon *cuts a chasm while ridges rise beyond.*

Stream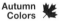

Autumn Colors

flow. Enter a flat, then come to the Big Devils Stairs Trail junction at 1.9 miles. ▶4

Turn right onto the Big Devils Stairs Trail, which follows the east rim of the gorge. Notice how abruptly the forest changes. The trees here are those typically found on drier south- or west-facing slopes—chestnut oak and Virginia pine—with an understory of mountain laurel. A scattering of pale white rock adds to the green mosaic. At 2.0 miles,

MILES

Big Devils Stairs Vista Elevation Profile

the declining path makes a few switchbacks while meandering down the rim of the gorge.

Ridgeline

Your descent may leave you antsy about finding the outcrop with the view, especially when boulders to the right of the trail through the woods seem to offer vantages. Stay with the trail and you won't miss the view. After an abrupt right turn, the trail comes to the edge of the gorge. Continue down the trail on stone steps, and descend to a large rock outcrop at 2.5 miles. ▶5 Grand views open of Big Devils Stairs canyon and the mountains beyond. Look at the stone walls rising from the stream below! Listen to the stream crashing through boulders at the canyon bottom. Follow the trail along the rim of the gorge for more vistas.

Great Views

Ahead, another outcrop hosts a gnarled pine hanging from its edge. Enjoy more views of the beautiful Shenandoah country, including Pignut Mountain, Piney Ridge, and fields beyond the park bounds. After this vista, the trail begins a steep descent and is not recommended. There is no public access from the lower end of the Big Devils Stairs. A trail once ran straight up the canyon, but after repeatedly washing out it was rerouted on the rim where you stand.

⊼ MILESTONES

▶ 1	0.0	Gravel Springs Gap Parking Area at milepost 17.6
▶ 2	0.4	Gravel Springs Hut
▶ 3	1.8	Cross stream of Big Devils Stairs canyon
▶ 4	1.9	Right on Big Devils Stairs Trail
▶ 5	2.5	Big Devils Stairs vista

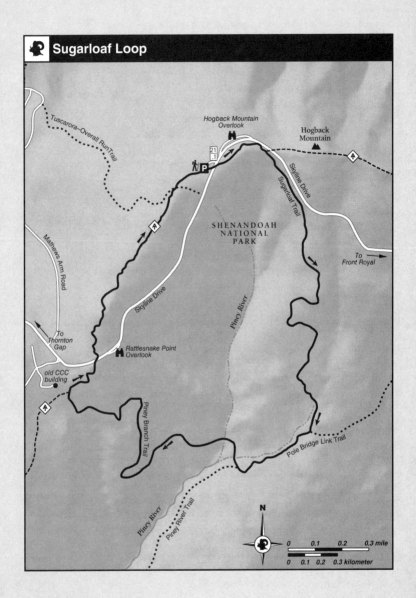

Sugarloaf Loop

Hogback Mountain Overlook

Hogback Mountain

Tuscarora–Overall RunTrail

21
1

Mathews Arm Road

Skyline Drive

Sugarloaf Trail

Skyline Drive

SHENANDOAH
NATIONAL
PARK

To
Front Royal

To
Thornton
Gap

Rattlesnake Point
Overlook

Piney River

old CCC
building

Piney Branch Trail

Pole Bridge Link Trail

Piney River

Piney River Trail

N

0   0.1   0.2   0.3 mile

0   0.1 0.2   0.3 kilometer

Sugarloaf Loop

This loop dips off the eastern side of Hogback Mountain into the upper Piney River Valley. You will relish far-reaching views on the Appalachian Trail (AT), then follow a moderate grade into the Piney River on the Sugarloaf Trail. A grassy flat beside the Piney River makes for a great resting spot. Head back to the high country, soaking in more great views from Hogback Mountain before completing the loop.

Best Time

Spring through fall are the most rewarding. Wildflowers bloom in the valley during spring. Summer offers a cool and shady respite. Enjoy views on clear fall days, and you might spot wildlife on the trail.

Finding the Trail

The hike starts at the parking area just south of the Hogback Mountain Overlook, milepost 21.1 on Skyline Drive. To reach the trailhead from the Thornton Gap Entrance Station, take Skyline Drive north for 10.4 miles to the parking area on the west side of Skyline Drive, just before Hogback Mountain Overlook. The loop hike starts on the eastern side of Skyline Drive where the AT crosses Skyline Drive.

Trail Description

From the parking area just south of Hogback Overlook, pick up the AT, northbound, as it crosses

TRAIL USE
Day Hiking,
Backpacking
LENGTH
4.7 miles, 3–4 hours
VERTICAL FEET
±870'
DIFFICULTY
– 1 2 **3** 4 5 +
TRAIL TYPE
Loop
START & FINISH
N38° 45.627'
W78° 16.953'

FEATURES
Ridgeline
Stream
Autumn Colors
Wildlife
Great Views
Geological Interest

FACILITIES
None

Surveying mountain lands *west from a trailside overlook on the Appalachian Trail*

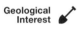

Geological Interest

over to the eastern side of Skyline Drive. ▶1 Hike through fern-floored oak woods, shortly climbing to a rocky knob spiked with uptilted rock. Note the rock combination to the right of the trail that resembles a chair. Many a hiker has had their picture taken in that oversized throne. At 0.2 mile, a side trail leads left to a rock outcrop framed in mountain ash trees. ▶2 The western vistas are extensive. Hogback Mountain Overlook is immediately below you. Overall Run cuts a chasm. Ridges rise around it. The Shenandoah Valley stretches out past

Sugarloaf Loop Elevation Profile

the park. Beyond the valley other mountains rise to frame the patchwork of farm, field, and town.

 Great Views

Descend among rocky woods. Notice how the winds have sculpted the trees to face easterly. Reach the slender Sugarloaf Trail at 0.3 mile. ▶3 Turn right onto a singletrack path lined with mountain laurel beneath scattered oaks. Briefly run parallel to Skyline Drive, joining an old wagon road. The Sugarloaf Trail curves back to the right, winding on a slightly sloped ridge, former pastureland. Descend to step over two rocky streamlets, wide but shallow feeder branches of the Piney River. Straight rock pioneer walls contrast with the fluid shapes of nature. Backpackers can find legal campsites off the trail in the next mile or so. This loop is a great break-in trip for the novice overnighter and a quick, quality one-night getaway for everyone.

Reach a trail junction at mile 1.7. Turn right onto the Pole Bridge Link Trail. ▶4 The land is level in these parts—for mountain land. It was cultivated too, despite the rocks you see. Pass through a changing forest, where hardwoods, such as black birch and yellow birch, are vying to replace the fallen hemlocks that once colored the vale evergreen. The gradual descent leads to another trail junction at 2.1 miles. Stay right with the Piney Branch Trail. ▶5

Step over the rocky branches you crossed earlier before reaching the upper Piney River in 0.1 mile. Large boulders and rocks line the watercourse. Cross the river to reach a grassy flat flanked by a large boulder. This locale makes a nice respite. A set of cascades downstream of this crossing are worth a look.

 Stream

Leave this low point of the loop—you are now a little higher than 2,500 feet—and start climbing toward the crest of the Blue Ridge on a gentle grade. Big rocks line the trailbed. At mile 3.2, pass through an open area with a tremendous rock face rising up the hill to your right. ▶6 In September, bears converge and eat cherries from trees that grow

 Geological Interest

Wildlife

nearby. You will see much purple, seed-laden bear scat along this path in the fall.

Curve uphill away from the roadbed to cross a second roadbed near a national park survey marker. The AT is just uphill, at 3.5 miles. Turn right onto the AT, making northbound tracks through open woodland where large widespread oaks grow over grass. ▶7 Younger trees vie for sunlight. Undulate over a rocky hill to reach Skyline Drive at 3.7 miles. ▶8 Rattlesnake Point Overlook is just up the road on your right. Keep northbound, crossing Skyline Drive, and ascend the south side of Hogback Mountain.

Ridgeline

A side trail at mile 4.0 leads left to an outcrop with views. ▶9 The ridgeline that is Massanutten Mountain forms a backdrop to South Fork Shenandoah River Valley. Range upon range of Shenandoah's mountains roll south. Dip into a pretty, grassy gap, then resume climbing to reach the Tuscarora–Overall Run Trail at mile 4.5. ▶10 Pass a limited vista point on trail right before drifting into the parking area at mile 4.7, completing your loop. ▶11

Great Views

𝝙	**MILESTONES**	
▶1	0.0	Parking area at milepost 21.1
▶2	0.2	View from Hogback Mountain
▶3	0.3	Right on Sugarloaf Trail
▶4	1.7	Right on Pole Bridge Link Trail
▶5	2.1	Stay right to join the Piney Branch Trail
▶6	3.2	Pass rock face
▶7	3.5	Right on the AT
▶8	3.7	Cross Skyline Drive
▶9	4.0	Vista
▶10	4.5	Tuscarora–Overall Run Trail leaves left
▶11	4.7	Parking area at milepost 21.1

Overall Run Falls

This there-and-back hike holds great rewards when you arrive—the park's highest falls and a grand vista beyond—and a warm-up fall along the way. And the trek is not too hard either. Start with a pleasant mountaintop stroll on the Appalachian Trail (AT), then wend your way down the slopes of Hogback Mountain, crossing many flats. Enter the Overall Run watershed. Pass Twin Falls, then come to Overall Run Falls. From a rocky precipice, you can see the nearby cataract and a whole lot more in the distance. Others will be enjoying the scenery with you, but it is not nearly as busy as Dark Hollow Falls and other cascades in the park's Central District. Nearby Mathews Arm Campground offers 217 campsites from May through October.

Best Time

Winter and early spring are the best times to see Shenandoah's highest falls. This locale also presents great views when the skies are clear, so keep that in mind.

Finding the Trail

The hike starts at the parking area just south of the Hogback Mountain Overlook, milepost 21.1 on Skyline Drive. To reach the trailhead from the Thornton Gap Entrance Station, take Skyline Drive north for 10.4 miles to the parking area on the west side of Skyline Drive, just before Hogback Mountain Overlook.

TRAIL USE
Day Hiking

LENGTH
6.8 miles, 4–5 hours

VERTICAL FEET
±1,500'

DIFFICULTY
– 1 2 3 **4** 5 +

TRAIL TYPE
Out-and-back

START & FINISH
N38° 45.627'
W78° 16.953'

FEATURES
Ridgeline
Stream
Waterfall
Autumn Colors
Wildflowers
Wildlife
Great Views
Geological Interest

FACILITIES
Campground nearby

SHENANDOAH
NATIONAL
PARK

Tuscarora–Overall Run Trail

Overall Run

Overall
Run Falls

Twin Falls

Beecher Ridge Trail

Heiskell Hollow Loop

Mathews Arm Trail

Bearwallow

Tuscarora–Overall Run Trail

Traces Trail

Mathews Arm
Campground

Hogback Mountain
Overlook

Hogback
Mountain

21
1

Skyline Drive

To
Thornton
Gap

To
Front Royal

N

0   0.1   0.2   0.3 mile

0   0.1 0.2   0.3 kilometer

Trail Description

Meet up with the AT as it skirts the south side of the parking area. ▶1 Turn right on the AT, heading southbound. You gently climb through lovely fern-carpeted woodland, passing a few rock outcrops. At a high point a spur leads left to jagged rocks and a limited view. Level off, then meet the Tuscarora–Overall Run Trail at 0.4 mile. ▶2 Turn right on the Tuscarora–Overall Run Trail. It proceeds downhill, snaking between rocks from which rise a rich forest. Rock and wood erosion bars cross the trail and form steps. Make a couple of switchbacks before coming to another trail junction at 1.1 miles. ▶3 Here, run into a connector to the Traces Trail. You aren't far from Mathews Arm Campground.

Turn right, staying on the Tuscarora–Overall Run Trail. At 1.2 miles, you pass a large embedded boulder on your left, then begin making your way down Hogback Mountain in stairstep fashion. The path will drop off, then level off, drop off again, and then level off once more. At 1.6 miles, step over the uppermost part of Overall Run. This trickling branch increases hope that there is a waterfall at the end of this thus-far-dry hike. These high-elevation flats seem to attract bears, which I have seen multiple times hereabouts. This area is shown on topo maps as "Bearwallow."

At 2.9 miles, the trail intersects the Mathews Arm Trail, which leaves left toward Mathews Arm Campground. Keep right. ▶4 Walk a short distance to another concrete signpost. Here, pass the now-abandoned section of Mathews Arm Trail. At this point you are likely wondering what water feeds the falls. The Tuscarora–Overall Run Trail answers the question, as you turn left down toward Overall Run on wood-and-earth steps. Reach the first cataract, Twin Falls, at 3.1 miles. ▶5

Ridgeline

Autumn Colors

This trek leads to the park's tallest cataract.

Wildlife

Stream

Wildflowers

Waterfall

Fern-carpeted woodland *borders the trail.*

A side trail leads left to the top of Twin Falls and a rock outcrop where you can view it. A large boulder splits Overall Run and divides the water, resulting in two streams dropping 29 feet. That is only the warm-up fall, but at least you are along and within earshot of moving water.

Overall Run Falls Elevation Profile

Keep astride the canyon, passing through laurel–oak woods. Tempting outcrops lure you to the edge of the valley, but they aren't the viewpoint. You will know it when you get there. Come to a wide-open cliff at 3.4 miles. ▶6

Geological Interest

The world opens beyond. To your left tumbles Overall Run Falls, at 93 feet the park's highest. The cataract drops over a huge rock face into the gorge below. More rock forms a wall on the far side of the falls. Nearby, other outcrops form vantage spots. The Overall Run canyon plunges below. It's a long way down there! The canyon maw divulges Page Valley and Massanutten Mountain in the backdrop. In the distance rise the Alleghenies and West Virginia—a great view overall and one of my favorites in the park.

Great Views

Waterfall

🚶	**MILESTONES**	
▶1	0.0	Parking area at milepost 21.1
▶2	0.4	Right on Tuscarora–Overall Run Trail
▶3	1.1	Stay right on Tuscarora–Overall Run Trail
▶4	2.9	Mathews Arm Trail leaves left
▶5	3.1	Twin Falls
▶6	3.4	Overall Run Falls

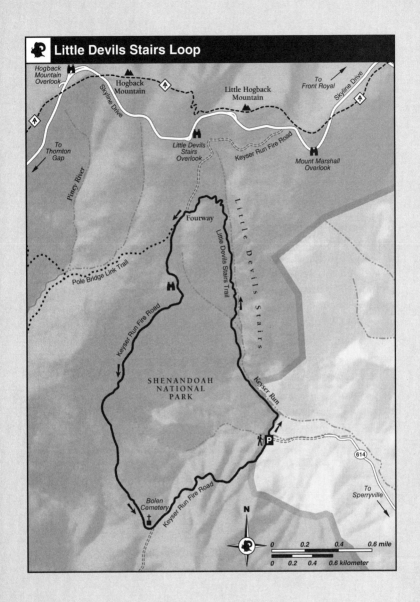

Little Devils Stairs Loop

Hogback Mountain Overlook

To Thornton Gap

Piney River

Skyline Drive

Hogback Mountain

Little Devils Stairs Overlook

Little Hogback Mountain

To Front Royal

Skyline Drive

Keyser Run Fire Road

Mount Marshall Overlook

Fourway

Little Devils Stairs

Little Devils Stairs Trail

Pole Bridge Link Trail

Keyser Run Fire Road

SHENANDOAH NATIONAL PARK

Keyser Run

P

614

To Sperryville

Bolen Cemetery

Keyser Run Fire Road

N

| 0 | 0.2 | 0.4 | 0.6 mile |
| 0 | 0.2 | 0.4 | 0.6 kilometer |

Little Devils Stairs Loop

This physically challenging but visually rewarding hike gives you something for every step you take. You undertake the challenging part (heading up Little Devils Stairs Canyon) at the beginning when you are fresh. The water, the rocks, the trees—there is beauty everywhere you look in this rough gorge. After emerging from the canyon, cruise down the mountains on Keyser Run Fire Road, taking in a well-earned vista and then passing pioneer internment Bolen Cemetery along the way.

Best Time

This hike requires multiple crossings of Keyser Run, at this point a smallish stream. Nonetheless, the crossings are easier from late-spring beyond into early winter. When the leaves are off, you can fully appreciate the rocky gorge of Little Devils Stairs.

Finding the Trail

From Thornton Gap, take US 211 east 7 miles to Sperryville. At a three-way intersection and the sign for the Sperryville Historic District, continue on US 211 east for 2.2 miles to VA 622, Gid Brown Hollow Road. Turn left on VA 622, and follow it for 1.9 miles to VA 614, Keyser Run Road. Turn left on VA 614, following it for 3.1 miles as it turns to gravel and ends at the Little Devils Stairs Parking Area. The Little Devils Stairs Trail leaves the right-hand side of the parking area.

TRAIL USE
Day Hiking,
Backpacking
LENGTH
5.4 miles, 3.5–4.5 hours
VERTICAL FEET
±1,390'
DIFFICULTY
– 1 2 3 **4** 5 +
TRAIL TYPE
Loop
START & FINISH
N38° 43.838'
W78° 15.491'

FEATURES
Ridgeline
Stream
Autumn Colors
Wildflowers
Great Views
Historical Interest
Geological Interest

FACILITIES
None

Trail Description

Leave the Little Devils Stairs Parking Area on the Little Devils Stairs Trail, and immediately step over two small streams. ▶1 Enter what once was a field in level woods. Notice the piles of rock, left over from when hardscrabble farmers squeezed out a life in this stony land.

Historical Interest

Stream

Wildflowers

Hike up a boulder-strewn canyon resembling the American West.

At 0.2 mile reach a gap alongside Keyser Run, which cuts the Little Devils Stairs Canyon. Turn left and begin to trace the creek upstream. At this point the grade is gentle, as the canyon hasn't closed yet. The footing is rocky. Large boulders are strewn about the hardwoods that shade the trail.

At 0.6 mile, the canyon closes in. Look for more pioneer walls. It's amazing to think pre-park Virginians lived in this sloped, nothing-but-stone vale that contrasts mightily with the fertile lands of the nearby Shenandoah Valley. But most of the people who resided in these parts preferred the mountain way of life and the trials that came with it, including the labor involved in building these rock walls.

At 0.9 mile, cross Keyser Run on the first of many crossings, all of which should be simple rock-hops at normal water levels. ▶2 Given the nature of Shenandoah's streams, Keyser Run is more rock than water, and it often fans into braids that flow

Little Devils Stairs Loop Elevation Profile

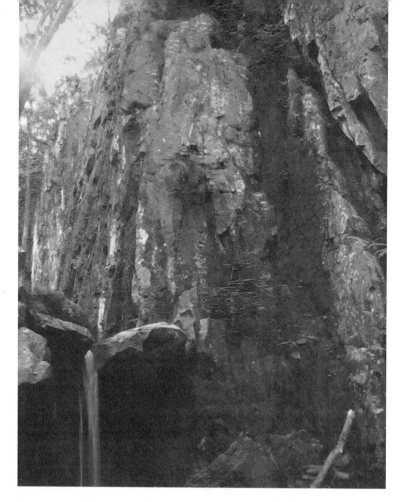

Keyser Run spills *between boulders against a sheer canyon wall backdrop.*

only during high-water events. The canyon narrows, and the forest of basswood, sycamore, and witch hazel becomes lush. Rock citadels rise to form canyon walls. Walk over, around, and among large boulders that litter the canyon floor. Beside you, the stream seeks its way down the gorge as fast as gravity allows.

 Geological Interest

Trail and creek merge time and again. The steep gradient of the stream creates occasional pools harboring trout and other aquatic life. The sheer walls of the canyon rise straight up above you. In other places scree slopes descend to the trail's edge. Tall and straight tulip trees grow on the rocky soil where they can gain purchase. Stinging nettles spread across the canyon floor where they can settle. The trail is very steep here and sometimes hard to follow through the rock jumbles. Stone steps aid hikers in places, but you will likely find places where occasional floods have undermined them. Watch for the blue blazes and keep going up.

Autumn Colors

At 1.4 miles, just after a crossing to the right-hand bank, you hike past a slide cascade that ends in a trailside plunge pool. The trail steepens. At mile 1.6, make your last crossing of Keyser Run, ending up on the left side of the gorge. ►3 Gently climb a series of switchbacks and level off, meeting the Keyser Run Fire Road at 2.0 miles. You have just climbed 1,500 feet. This trail junction is known as Fourway.

Waterfall

At 2.2 miles, turn left on the Keyser Run Fire Road, and begin a trifling descent after your rigorous climb through the rigorous canyon. ►4 Trailside hardwoods only partially canopy the track. Enjoy the forest around you, breathing easy. Funny thing about the fire road: it was once known as Jinney Gray Fire Road, but after her history was lost to time, the park service changed the name to Keyser Run Fire Road. In summer wildflowers color the edges of the track, and ripe berries tempt the hiker.

Great Views

At 2.5 miles, a spur trail leads left to a rock outcrop and vista. ►5 Here, you can look into the canyon below as well as out at waves of mountains beyond and the crest of the Blue Ridge. Watch for a small rocked-in spring branch at 3.1 miles. At other times, small seeps spill over the trail. Pass under a transmission line at 3.8 miles. Enter a deep woods flat dominated by white pine and some large-for-the-species sassafras trees. Watch for rock fence lines and larger trees of old-home sites.

Arrive at Bolen Cemetery at 4.3 miles. The well-tended internment is lined with maples and surrounded by a rock wall. The graves range from carved marble to simple fieldstones. Just beyond, the Hull School Trail leaves right. Stay left on Keyser Run Fire Road, and descend beneath more white pines. ▶6 Watch for more rock walls and the old pre-park road running parallel to the modern fire road. Pass around a pole gate at 5.2 miles. Keep left, and complete your loop at mile 5.4. ▶7

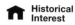
Historical Interest

𝕏 MILESTONES

▶	1	0.0	Little Devils Stairs Trailhead
▶	2	0.9	First crossing of Keyser Run
▶	3	1.6	Last crossing of Keyser Run
▶	4	2.2	Left on Keyser Run Fire Road
▶	5	2.5	Vista
▶	6	4.3	Left just after Bolen Cemetery
▶	7	5.4	Little Devils Stairs Trailhead

Tuscarora Trail

Thompson Hollow Trail

Beecher–Overall Connector Trail

Overall Run

Tuscarora–Overall Run Trail

N

0   0.2   0.4   0.6 mile

0   0.2   0.4   0.6 kilometer

SHENANDOAH
NATIONAL
PARK

Overall
Run Falls

Twin Falls

Beecher Ridge Trail

B e e c h e r   R i d g e

Heiskell Hollow Trail

Dry Run

Compton Hollow

Weddlewood Trail

Mathews Arm Trail

Tuscarora–Overall Run Trail

Traces Trail

Mathews Arm Campground

Traces Connector

Knob Mountain Trail

K n o b   M o u n t a i n

Jeremys Run

Elkwallow Trail

Skyline Drive

Mathews Arm Road

22
.2

To
Front Royal

Knob Mountain
Cutoff Trail

Jeremys Run Trail

To
Thornton
Gap

Overall Run Loop

Leave the kids behind on this challenging loop that is a personal favorite. Beyond its high point near Mathews Arm Campground, the hike drops more than 2,000 feet, and then climbs back up, every foot. Leave near the Mathews Arm Campground entrance station. Circle the campground before joining remote Beecher Ridge, making a glorious walk through lush forests and parklike woodlands before dropping to Overall Run. The lower part of Overall Run reveals its former pioneer presence. Work upstream in a rugged gorge, passing a superlative swimming hole. The gorge tightens and narrows, and the stream is forced to drop over a series of falls into more large pools. Come to Overall Run Falls, the park's highest at 93 feet. You can observe this cataract and enjoy a mountain panorama before making your way back to the trailhead.

TRAIL USE
Day Hiking,
Backpacking
LENGTH
9.2 miles, 5.5–7 hours
VERTICAL FEET
±2,060'
DIFFICULTY
– 1 2 3 4 **5** +
TRAIL TYPE
Loop
START & FINISH
N38° 45.640'
W78° 17.899'

FEATURES
Ridgeline
Stream
Waterfall
Autumn Colors
Wildlife
Great Views
Swimming
Secluded
Steep
Historical Interest
Geological Interest

FACILITIES
Campground nearby

Best Time

This hike is best done when nearby Mathews Arm Campground is open, generally mid-May–October. Otherwise you have to walk the campground access road from Skyline Drive to get to the trail. The crossings of Overall Run will be easier then as well.

Finding the Trail

From milepost 22.2 on Skyline Drive, follow the entrance road from Skyline Drive for 0.6 mile into Mathews Arm Campground. When you reach a T-intersection just after the campground entrance

station, turn right and then immediately right again
into a large parking area.

Trail Description

The Traces Nature Trail has two entrances from the
trailhead parking area—make sure to take the Traces
Nature Trail that leaves from the T-intersection near
the campground entrance station rather than the
one that leads directly from the trailhead parking
area near the campground amphitheater. ►1 On
the proper segment of the Traces Nature Trail, you
immediately pass under a power line, then roll in
rocky highland woods.

Meet the Mathews Arm Trail at 0.6 mile. ►2
Turn left here on a wide, roadlike track, descending to pass a closing meadow on your right. Look
for deer here; you may well see one in the morning or evening. Pass the Weddlewood Trail at 0.9
mile. The wide roadbed makes for easy walking,
but the Mathews Arm Trail soon narrows to meet
the Beecher Ridge Trail at 1.4 miles. Turn left here,
joining this lesser-trod path. ►3 Enter a remote section of the park. Singletrack Beecher Ridge Trail
descends in oak-dominated woods. The valley of
Overall Run falls away to your right. This trail is
heavily traveled by bears—you will likely see bear
scat on the path in summer. Join the crest of wide

Wildlife

Ridgeline

Secluded

Overall Run Loop Elevation Profile

Beecher Ridge at 2.2 miles. Level off in parklike woodland at 2.4 miles. Enjoy the forest cruise as you skim an inconsequential knob. Notice the still-standing locust trees here—many are beginning to fall in inevitable forest succession. Hickories and oaks, shaded by the locusts, are taking over, and the locust trees, notoriously rot-resistant, will eventually decay back into the earth, feeding the future mighty oaks and hickories.

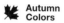 **Autumn Colors**

Resume a rapid descent amid oak-laden rocky woods with little ground cover. The ridgeline narrows. Pines join the fray before making a trail junction at 3.7 miles. Turn right toward Overall Run on the Beecher-Overall Connector Trail. ▶4 Keep going forward, curving north on a dry ridge widespread with blueberry bushes. The woods thicken when you enter the Overall Run valley. Reach Overall Run at 4.2 miles. ▶5 Here the stream is braided and is more rock than water, perhaps even entirely dry, in summer and fall. Following rains it can be torrential. If it is, do not attempt to cross it. Continue stepping across several stream braids, making the north side of the run.

At 4.3 miles, turn right at a concrete marker post, joining an old roadbed heading easterly, officially on the Tuscarora–Overall Run Trail. Note the rock walls in this wide valley, evidence of former settlements and hardscrabble farming in this stony soil, now supporting white pines. Buckled rock walls constrict the valley at 4.8 miles. In high water the whole stream funnels through this portal.

 Historical Interest

 Stream

The trail climbs away from the stream, and at 4.9 miles, you reach a potentially confusing four-way junction. ▶6 To your left is a campsite. The blue-blazed Tuscarora–Overall Run Trail keeps straight, and to your right, a trail leads to a sunny outcrop and a surprisingly deep swimming hole below a rock slab cascade. This is a special area. Please treat it with care. The open outcrop is great

 Swimming

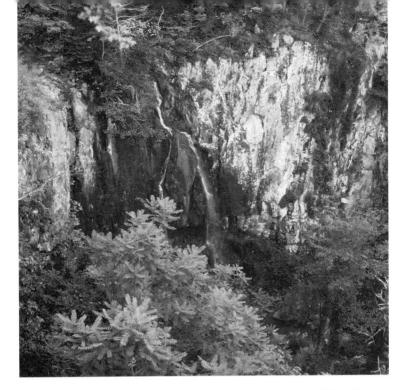

Big Falls, *the park's highest cataract at 93 feet, also goes by the name Overall Run Falls.*

for drying off after a dip in the crystalline pool. The hike continues climbing to shortly meet the Thompson Hollow Trail, which leads left to the park boundary. ▶7

Keep making your way up the scenic gorge, pocked with spicebush and pawpaw, on a very rocky track that slows your progress. Cross Overall Run at 5.6 and 6.0 miles. The trail becomes very steep as you leave the creek at 6.3 miles, switchbacking toward the canyon rim. ▶8 At 6.6 miles, a spur trail leads right to a cliff that many hikers bypass. ▶9 You can look up toward an outcrop you will soon be standing on. Make the rim and reach another cliff with a fantastic view at 7.2 miles. ▶10 Across the gorge is Overall Run Falls, the park's highest at 93 feet. In winter, the fall may be frozen over the entire rock face. In summer, flow can be low and sluggish. Below, Overall Run Canyon winds its way

Steep

Geological Interest

Waterfall

toward the Page Valley. Beyond stands Massanutten Mountain. Beyond that rise the Alleghenies.

Continue up the rim, and soon pass wooded Twin Falls to your right, a much smaller drop at 29 feet. You have to go off the trail a little to get a good view. The path switchbacks away from the creek and comes to a concrete post and the Mathews Arm Trail at 7.4 miles. Stay right here and just ahead the Tuscarora–Overall Run Trail leaves left for the AT. ▶11 Stay right with the Mathews Arm Trail, making a gentle uptick to reach the Beecher Ridge Trail at 7.8 miles. ▶12 From here, make a 1.4-mile backtrack to the trailhead. ▶13

 Great Views

Waterfall

🚶	MILESTONES	
▶1	0.0	Traces Nature Trail parking
▶2	0.6	Left on Mathews Arm Trail
▶3	1.4	Left on Beecher Ridge Trail
▶4	3.7	Right on Beecher-Overall Connector Trail
▶5	4.2	Right on Tuscarora–Overall Run Trail after crossing Overall Run
▶6	4.9	Swimming hole on right
▶7	5.0	Thompson Hollow Trail leaves left
▶8	6.3	Leave creek
▶9	6.6	Spur to cliff
▶10	7.2	Overall Run Falls and Page Valley vista
▶11	7.4	Right with Mathews Arm Trail
▶12	7.8	Pass Beecher Ridge Trail
▶13	9.2	Traces Nature Trail parking

Heiskell Hollow Loop

SHENANDOAH
NATIONAL
PARK

Beecher–Overall Connector Trail

Tuscarora Trail

Thompson Hollow Trail

Tuscarora–Overall Run Trail

Overall Run

Overall Run Falls

Twin Falls

Beecher Ridge Trail

B e e c h e r R i d g e

Dry Run

Heiskell Hollow Trail

Compton Hollow

Waddlewood Trail

Mathews Arm Trail

Traces Trail

Tuscarora–Overall Run Trail

Mathews Arm Campground

Traces Connector

Mathews Arm Road

K n o b   M o u n t a i n

Knob Mountain Trail

Jeremys Run

Elkwallow Trail

Skyline Drive

22.2

To Front Royal

Knob Mountain Cutoff Trail

Jeremys Run Trail

To Thornton Gap

N

0   0.2   0.4   0.6 mile

0   0.2   0.4   0.6 kilometer

Heiskell Hollow Loop

This hike explores the least-visited ridge and valley of the greater Mathews Arm area of the park, and is one of the least-hiked quality circuits in the park. It has no single superlative feature to draw hikers in but offers you a chance to explore the park in solitude. First, circle around Mathews Arm Campground on the Traces Nature Trail, eventually reaching secluded Beecher Ridge. Travel the spine of this regally forested highland before picking up the Heiskell Hollow Trail. Dip into the East Fork Valley before winding your way up Keyser Hollow and back onto Mathews Arm. Plenty of pioneer evidence awaits a sharp-eyed hiker.

TRAIL USE
Day Hiking,
Backpacking
LENGTH
7.2 miles, 4–5 hours
VERTICAL FEET
±1,620'
DIFFICULTY
– 1 2 3 **4** 5 +
TRAIL TYPE
Loop
START & FINISH
N38° 45.640'
W78° 17.899'

Best Time

This hike is best done when nearby Mathews Arm Campground is open, generally mid-May–October. Otherwise you have to walk the campground access road from Skyline Drive to get to the trail.

Finding the Trail

From milepost 22.2 on Skyline Drive, follow the entrance road from Skyline Drive for 0.6 mile into Mathews Arm Campground. When you reach a T-intersection just after the campground entrance station, turn right and then immediately right again into a large parking area.

FEATURES
Ridgeline
Stream
Autumn Colors
Wildflowers
Wildlife
Secluded
Historical Interest

FACILITIES
Campground nearby

Trail Description

Start your loop on the Traces Nature Trail. ►1 Be careful because it has two entrances from the trailhead parking area. Make sure to pick up the Traces Nature Trail that leaves from the T-intersection near the campground entrance station rather than the one that leads directly from the trailhead parking area near the campground amphitheater. Once you are on the proper segment of the Traces Nature Trail, you immediately pass under a power line, then undulate in rocky highland woods.

Come to Mathews Arm Trail at 0.6 mile. Turn right here. ►2 Pass a small field where deer may be seen browsing. The Weddlewood Trail leaves left at 0.9 mile. Keep straight on the wide Mathews Arm Trail. The wide roadbed makes for easy walking, but the Mathews Arm Trail narrows before coming to Beecher Ridge Trail at 1.4 miles. Turn left here. ►3 The faint-but-clear trail attests to the solitude found along its length.Tall oaks shade singletrack Beecher Ridge Trail. The valley of Overall Run falls away to your right and East Fork to your left. It seems bears use the trail more than people—you will likely see bear scat on the path in summer.

Join the crest of wide Beecher Ridge at 2.2 miles. Level off in parklike woodland at 2.4 miles. Resume a rapid descent amid oak-laden rocky woods with

Solitude lovers will enjoy this circuit.

Wildlife

Ridgeline ▲

Secluded

Heiskell Hollow Loop Elevation Profile

little ground cover. The ridgeline narrows. Pines mix in with the oaks.

Come to a forlorn trail junction at 3.7 miles. ▶4 Stay left at the intersection, still on Beecher Ridge Trail. Wander southeasterly through pine–oak woods. Watch for old pioneer roads crossing Heiskell Hollow Trail. Dip to a dry streambed, climb a bit, then resume your quest for East Fork. Reach East Fork at 4.4 miles. Traverse a rocky area dividing East Fork from Moody Creek, coming to the Heiskell Hollow Trail at 4.5 miles. ▶5 Turn left here, ascending along Moody Creek in Keyser Hollow. Angle up a mountainside in piney woods with a grassy understory. Meet the Weddlewood Trail at 6.2 miles. ▶6 Stay with Heiskell Hollow Trail, ascending through open, rock-strewn forest escorted by rock walls. Watch for old roads splintering off the path. Also look for large oaks, which have grown tall above the rocky floor. Emerge onto the crumbling asphalt of the access road for Mathews Arm water treatment station at 6.8 miles. Turn left, ascending a wide track. ▶7 Come out near Mathews Arm Campground entrance station at 7.2 miles, completing your loop. ▶8

 Secluded

 Stream

Wildflowers

 Historical Interest

🚶	**MILESTONES**	
▶ 1	0.0	Traces Nature Trail parking (Mathews Arm Campground entrance)
▶ 2	0.6	Right on Mathews Arm Trail
▶ 3	1.4	Left on Beecher Ridge Trail
▶ 4	3.7	Stay left at intersection, still on Beecher Ridge Trail
▶ 5	4.5	Left on Heiskell Hollow Trail
▶ 6	6.2	Pass Weddlewood Trail
▶ 7	6.8	Left on crumbling asphalt road
▶ 8	7.2	Traces Nature Trail parking (Mathews Arm Campground entrance)

Elkwallow Loop

To Front Royal

Rattlesnake Point Overlook

Traces Connector

Mathews Arm Road

Mathews Arm Trail

Mathews Arm Campground

Traces Trail

Traces Trail

Piney Branch Trail

Piney River

Piney River Trail

old CCC building

Range View Cabin

Piney Ridge Trail

Skyline Drive

Elkwallow Trail

Heiskell Hollow Trail

Knob Mountain Trail

Jeremys Run

SHENANDOAH NATIONAL PARK

Elkwallow Gap

To Thorton Gap

Elkwallow Picnic Ground

Knob Mountain Cutoff Trail

Jeremys Run Trail

Jeremys Run

Knob Mountain Trail

Knob Mountain

0.6 mile

0.4

0.6 kilometer

0.2   0.4

0   0.2

N

Elkwallow Loop

It's a wonder that this classic Shenandoah circuit hike isn't done more, considering the proximity of camping and other national park facilities to the often-level loop. First, leave the Mathews Arm Campground on the Elkwallow Trail. It navigates boulders galore before settling down and making a pleasantly level highland track on the west side of the Blue Ridge. The loop joins the Appalachian Trail (AT) near Elkwallow Wayside, where food and other supplies are available. Pass a picnic area and spring before joining Jeremys Run Trail, dipping to Jeremys Run. Cross the fine mountain stream then climb a stony slope, joining the seldom-trod Knob Mountain Trail. This path offers everywhere-you-look beauty on a remarkably level track, allowing you to enjoy the national park scenery. The final ascent leads back to Mathews Arm Campground.

Best Time

This hike is best done when nearby Mathews Arm Campground is open, generally mid-May–October. Otherwise you have to walk the campground access road from Skyline Drive to get to the trail.

Finding the Trail

From milepost 22.2 on Skyline Drive, follow the entrance road for 0.6 mile from Skyline Drive into Mathews Arm Campground, reaching a T-intersection just after the campground entrance station. Turn right here, then immediately turn right again into a large parking area. The Elkwallow Trail

TRAIL USE
Day Hiking
LENGTH
5.6 miles, 3–4 hours
VERTICAL FEET
±825'
DIFFICULTY
– 1 2 **3** 4 5 +
TRAIL TYPE
Loop
START & FINISH
N38° 45.604'
W78° 17.871'

FEATURES
Ridgeline
Stream
Autumn Colors
Wildflowers
Wildlife
Secluded

FACILITIES
Campground and
camp store
Picnic area

Asters glow *in the autumn sun.*

starts across the campground access road from the parking area, near the entrance station (driving in, you can see the Elkwallow Trail on your left, just before coming to the campground entrance station).

Trail Description

Turn left onto the Elkwallow Trail ▶1 as it briefly follows a grassy road then splits right as a single-track path heading downhill in a rocky hardwood forest of witch hazel, white oak, and fire cherry.

Elkwallow Loop Elevation Profile

Drop off a stone bluff to reach a high-elevation wet-land. A long boardwalk, rare for this mountain park, spans these headwaters of Jeremys Run. Continue on the level as Jeremys Run falls away below. This easy walking allows you to observe the forest comprehensively. The woodlands of Shenandoah National Park have been in a near continual state of change since the park's inception. First, the cleared pastures of pre-park settlers began the slow process of succession from field to forest. Later, the gypsy moth came in and decimated the mighty oaks of Shenandoah, setting off another chain reaction of reforestation where the oaks fell. Lately, the demise of the hemlock has shaped the woodland. Once again opportunistic plants are coming in and rising where hemlocks once stood.

 Stream

 Wildflowers

In winter, views open to your right. Pass an obvious trailside boulder at 1.2 miles. The next mile or so is a good place to spot deer; the open forest and adjacent clearings lure them in. Come near Skyline Drive, and then intersect the AT at 1.8 miles. Turn right here, ▶2 southbound on Shenandoah's master path. (Elkwallow Wayside is just ahead if you keep straight on the Elkwallow Trail. The wayside offers drinks, food, and camping supplies in season.) The AT meanders downhill in slightly sloped forest with little understory. At 2.1 miles, turn right with the AT, as a spur trail leads left to Elkwallow Picnic Ground. ▶3 Soon pass a spring used by AT hikers, near which the long-dismantled Elkwallow Shelter once stood.

At 2.3 miles, leave the AT, joining the Jeremys Run Trail. ▶4 Work downhill, entering the Jeremys Run Valley. Come to Jeremys Run and a trail inter-section at 3.1 miles. Turn right here on the Knob Mountain Cutoff Trail to immediately walk across clear Jeremys Run on stones. Now comes the only hard part of the hike—a 350-foot climb in a half mile. Angle up the south slope of Knob Mountain.

 Wildflowers

▶5 Pass several partially open stone slabs on your switchback ascent amid hickories.

At 3.6 miles, turn right onto the Knob Mountain Trail, making another, milder climb on a wide track. ▶6 Level off at 3.9 miles, then make a glorious ridgeline walk. Sturdy white oaks and white pines shade the path. Watch for bears in the flats. Rocks have been cleared from the remarkably flat trail.

Ridgeline ▲

Wildlife 🦌

At 5.1 miles, reach a service road for the campground water treatment plant. Turn right on the crumbly asphalt, toward the campground. ▶7 Soon pass the Heiskell Hollow Trail. Ahead, pass around a chain gate, and emerge on blacktop near the campground entrance station, completing your hike at 5.6 miles. ▶8

🚶 MILESTONES

▶	1	0.0	Elkwallow Trailhead near Mathews Arm entrance station
▶	2	1.8	Right on Appalachian Trail
▶	3	2.1	Spur leads left to Elkwallow Picnic Ground
▶	4	2.3	Right on Jeremys Run Trail
▶	5	3.1	Right on Knob Mountain Cutoff Trail
▶	6	3.6	Right on Knob Mountain Trail
▶	7	5.1	Right on asphalt service road
▶	8	5.6	End of hike near campground entrance station

Piney River Falls

It's surprising that this hike isn't more popular. The scenery along the way meets high Shenandoah standards, and the falls are a worthy destination. To get there, leave the high country, and gently wind your way through eye-pleasing, high-country woods. Work your way down through the Piney River Valley on old roads, and take a short side trail to the three-tier falls. It's a good way to spend an afternoon.

Best Time

The lesser-visited destination offers solitude most of the year. In spring it offers a bold watercourse and wildflowers. Summer is cool along the river. Fall has color. If you want maximum solitude, take this hike in winter.

Finding the Trail

From the Thornton Gap Entrance Station, take Skyline Drive north for 9.4 miles to the old Civilian Conservation Corps (CCC) building in the upper Piney River area. The entrance road is on your right at milepost 22.1, just north of the turn to Mathews Arm Campground on the left. Park in the designated visitor parking area across from the CCC building. The Piney Branch Trail starts between the parking area and Skyline Drive.

TRAIL USE
Day Hiking,
Backpacking
LENGTH
6.8 miles, 3.5–4.5 hours
VERTICAL FEET
±1,325'
DIFFICULTY
– 1 2 3 **4** 5 +
TRAIL TYPE
Out-and-back
START & FINISH
N38° 45.037'
W78° 17.599'

FEATURES
Ridgeline
Stream
Waterfall
Autumn Colors
Wildflowers
Secluded

FACILITIES
None

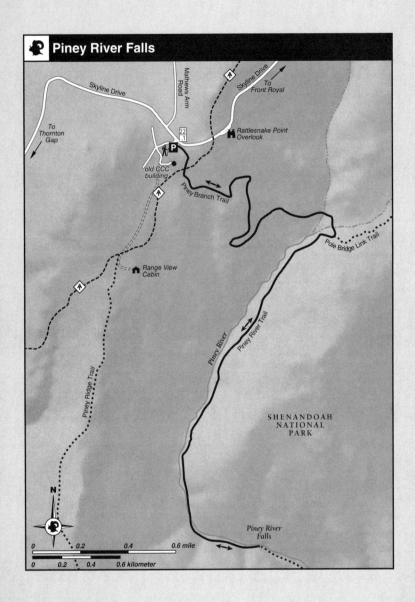

Piney River Falls

Skyline Drive

Mathews Arm Road

Skyline Drive
To Front Royal

To Thornton Gap

22
1

P

old CCC building

Rattlesnake Point Overlook

Piney Branch Trail

Pole Bridge Link Trail

Range View Cabin

Piney River

Piney River Trail

Piney Ridge Trail

SHENANDOAH NATIONAL PARK

N

Piney River Falls

0   0.2   0.4   0.6 mile

0   0.2   0.4   0.6 kilometer

Trail Description

Start your hike at the back of the field between
Skyline Drive and the parking area across from the
old CCC camp building. ▶1 Look for the concrete
post marked PINEY BRANCH TRAIL. Begin walking through a forest of black locust trees that are
repopulating what once was pasture. Up to a third
of the land within the park was once field, pasture,
or meadow—treeless. Even now the trees continue
to inexorably reclaim former farm country, which
was once woods even farther back in time. At 0.1
mile intersect the Appalachian Trail (AT) and continue straight on a track much fainter than the AT.
Note the apple trees in the area.

The Piney Branch Trail winds its way down to
the valley, making very gentle, loping switchbacks.
Pass by an open rock slab at 0.4 mile, then a wooded
boulder field. The less windswept forest is much
taller here than it is near the trailhead. The old roadbed comes to the upper reaches of the Piney River
at mile 1.3. ▶2 Big boulders line the small river. The
grassy area beside the stream makes for a good place
to relax. Curve right away from Piney River, crossing spring branches flowing between rocks. Park
personnel did an outstanding job designing a dry
track through this mushy area. The trail meets the
Pole Bridge Link Trail at 1.5 miles. ▶3

Turn right, staying with the now-narrower and
even lesser-used section of the Piney Branch Trail.
Wildflowers thrive in the Piney River Valley. The
mountain laurel–lined path follows an old road on
a slight downgrade. The gorge of Piney River cuts
ever deeper to your right. At mile 2.0, the old road
continues straight, but the Piney Branch Trail veers
right and follows another old road. The trail runs a
fair distance above the creek, descending at a moderate but steady clip.

At 2.7 miles, the trail comes very close to Piney
River. ▶4 A spur trail leads right to the riverside

This is one of the
most undervisited and
underappreciated falls
in the park.

▲ Ridgeline

⚡ Stream

❗ Secluded

✿ Wildflowers

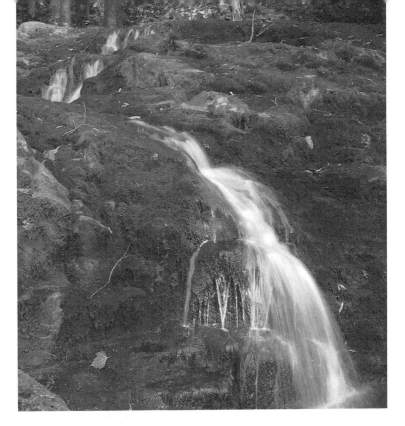

Piney River Falls *tumbles 25 feet into a pool.*

and a pleasant picnic spot. Continue along the waterway, appreciating its pools and shoals, in a wildflower-filled flat, where big boulders pock the rising hillside.

Piney River Falls Elevation Profile

Cross the Piney River at 3.0 miles. ►5 This is a rock-hop at normal flows and may take a little fancy footwork. Another method is to shed your shoes and socks and walk through the water with a stout stick as an aid. At lower levels this crossing is a breeze. You are now on the southern side of the river, and the falls are only 0.4 mile away. Watch and listen for other cascades along Piney River while making your way downstream. Cove hardwoods of yellow birch, black birch, red maple, and basswood shade the frothing watercourse.

 Stream

Stumble through river rubble, rocks strewn here from high-water events. Ferns spread wide beside rock outcrops. Sycamores find their place amid the rocks and water. Pass two house-sized rock bluffs on your right at mile 3.2 in this rugged gorge. A hard-to-reach 10-foot, two-tier waterfall spills to your left. Begin listening for Piney River Falls, only 0.2 mile away. At mile 3.4, turn left on a side trail leading to the cataract. ►6 Piney River Falls is a 25-foot, triple-tiered cascade coursing over mossy rock into a deep and wide pool. Rock slabs border much of the drop and make for good observation locales. It's a good place to cool off after a hot hike. Relax a spell.

 Waterfall

🚶 MILESTONES

► 1	0.0	Old CCC building at milepost 22.1
► 2	1.3	Cross Piney River
► 3	1.5	Stay right with Piney Branch Trail
► 4	2.7	Come back along Piney River
► 5	3.0	Cross Piney River
► 6	3.4	Piney River Falls

Knob Mountain and Jeremys Run Loop

Piney Ridge Trail

Elkwallow Gap

Skyline Drive

To Front Royal

Elkwallow Wayside

Elkwallow Picnic Ground

Knob Mountain Cutoff Trail

Knob Mountain Trail

24

SHENANDOAH NATIONAL PARK

To Thornton Gap

B l u e   R i d g e

Jeremys Run

Jeremys Run Trail

Skyline Drive

K n o b   M o u n t a i n

Knob Mountain Trail

Moody Creek

Beahm Lane

Jeremys Run

Neighbor Mountain Trail

Vaughn Summit Road

N

0   0.5   1.0   1.5 miles

0   0.5   1.0   1.5 kilometers

Knob Mountain and Jeremys Run Loop

This is a long and rewarding loop exploring points high and low. Leave Elkwallow Picnic Ground (which has water, restrooms, and shaded tables), dropping to upper Jeremys Run, one of the park's biggest, wildest valleys. Climb to Knob Mountain, then traverse its ridgeline, enjoying views on the way to Jeremys Run. Make your way up gorgeous Jeremys Run valley, crossing the stream more than a dozen times. Watch for brook trout in the deep pools of Jeremys Run. You may want to cool off in the stream while down there. Leave the valley, backtracking to Elkwallow Picnic Ground. Don't expect to have company on Knob Mountain, though you may see a few people along Jeremys Run.

Best Time

This is a great summertime hike. You can cruise the high country, and just when things get a little hot, the trek takes you along the pools of Jeremys Run, ideal for fishing or swimming. Fall is good too, since the low stream will make the 16 crossings easier. Conversely, Jeremys Run may be too high during winter and early spring.

Finding the Trail

From Thornton Gap, take Skyline Drive north for 7.4 miles to Elkwallow Picnic Ground at milepost 24.1. Drive to the low end of the picnic area and park. The spur trail to the Appalachian Trail (AT) leaves here. The Elkwallow Wayside, a short distance north on Skyline Drive, has a camp store and

TRAIL USE
Day Hiking,
Backpacking

LENGTH
13.1 miles,
8.5–9.5 hours

VERTICAL FEET
±1,770'

DIFFICULTY
– 1 2 3 4 **5** +

TRAIL TYPE
Loop

START & FINISH
N38° 45.715'
W78° 18.295'

FEATURES
Summit
Ridgeline
Stream
Waterfall
Autumn Colors
Wildlife
Great Views
Swimming
Secluded
Steep
Geological Interest

FACILITIES
Camp store (in season)
Picnic area with water
and restrooms

Jeremys Run *has clear, cool pools that harbor brook trout.*

Knob Mountain and Jeremys Run Loop Elevation Profile

food offerings during the warm season if you don't feel like picnicking.

Trail Description

Start your loop on the spur trail leaving Elkwallow Picnic Ground. ►1 Leave Elkwallow, and in fifty yards intersect the AT. Stay left, heading downhill, southbound through woods. On your left pass Elkwallow Spring, which serves up chilly water even on the hottest summer day. Meet the Jeremys Run Trail at 0.2 mile. ►2 Keep straight on the Jeremys Run Trail, as the AT makes a hard left here. Travel a long-abandoned roadbed on surprisingly level terrain. Shortly switchback downhill, crossing the outflow of the aforementioned spring. The trail takes you parallel to Jeremys Run, heading deeper into its valley. At 1.0 mile, meet the Knob Mountain Cutoff Trail, and begin the loop portion of the hike. ►3 Turn right on the Knob Mountain Cutoff Trail. Immediately rock-hop Jeremys Run. Get water here since there is none for miles along Knob Mountain.

After crossing Jeremys Run, the trail switchbacks up a piney, rocky slope. The steep path makes use of a few old roads. Level off and come to the Knob Mountain Trail at 1.6 miles. ►4 Turn left, west, on the Knob Mountain Trail, following a former fire road. Here, the trail undulates over small prominences and outcrops, then dips to gaps, climbing ever so slightly toward the Knob Mountain summit. Views of the Shenandoah Valley are off to your right. The valley of Jeremys Run falls off to your left.

The trail is only partly canopied and often bordered with brush, including blackberries in summer. By mile 3.0, the ridge has become wide and level. This is grouse country; don't be surprised if a brown fowl flutters away at your feet. Just before reaching the summit, the former fire road ends at

This hike presents both streamside and mountaintop highlights.

 Stream

 Steep

 Ridgeline

Summit ▲ a concrete post. Continue forward on a footpath, making an abrupt ascent to the summit (2,865') at 3.9 miles, which also has a concrete post. ▶5

The trail drops sharply off the summit. Look for the town of Luray and for Massanutten Mountain through the trees while working your way toward Jeremys Run. The path makes repeated switchbacks on the ridge. At 4.6 miles, the trail splits a gap and traces the left side of the ridge. Jeremys Run flows below you, and Neighbor Mountain rises across the valley. More switchbacks lead you through an area of pine trees and abundant views **Great Views** of the Shenandoah Valley. Pass a spring on your right at 6.0 miles. ▶6 It has been rocked in but may still need to be cleaned out.

Great Views

Neighbor Mountain looms larger as you continue descending. Soon you can hear the intonations of Jeremys Run. At mile 6.7, pass a pioneer fenceline and spring. Come to your first crossing of Jeremys Run at the head of a pretty pool, then intersect the **Stream** Jeremys Run Trail at 7.1 miles. ▶7 Turn left and just ahead is the Neighbor Mountain Trail junction. Here are some good sitting rocks for a break.

Start up Jeremys Run Trail on a mild grade. Stone walls line the path. Regal white pines grow on former fields. Sycamores shade the stream, where brook trout gather in deep pools that double as places for sweaty hikers to cool off.

When rock bluffs crowd the stream, the trail crosses to the other side toward flatter terrain. Your next crossing is at 7.4 miles. This pattern continues time and again up the valley. These fords are dangerous only in times of high water. Most of the time you can make it dry-shod. The stream sometimes braids into dry channels. While walking up the **Waterfall** valley, you are often 10–20 feet above the stream, allowing for good looks into the watercourse. Pass a 10-foot, two-tier waterfall and popular swimming **Swimming** hole at 7.8 miles. ▶8

Cross the run at 8.4 miles and then again at 9.2 and 9.5 miles. After 9.9 miles, the crossings become more frequent. A total of 16 crossings, including the first one at the lower end of the Knob Mountain Trail, bring you to the head of the valley and the junction with the Knob Mountain Cutoff Trail at mile 12.1. ►9 Retrace your steps up the Jeremys Run Trail, coming once again to the AT. Head up the AT for 0.2 mile, then veer right up to the Elkwallow Picnic Ground, completing your loop at 13.1 miles. ►10

🚶	**MILESTONES**	
►1	0.0	Elkwallow Picnic Ground at milepost 24.1
►2	0.2	Pick up Jeremys Run Trail
►3	1.0	Right on Knob Mountain Cutoff Trail
►4	1.6	Left on Knob Mountain Trail
►5	3.9	Knob Mountain summit
►6	6.0	Spring to right of trail
►7	7.1	Left on Jeremys Run Trail
►8	7.8	Waterfall and swimming hole
►9	12.1	Knob Mountain Cutoff Trail leaves left
►10	13.1	Elkwallow Picnic Ground at milepost 24.1

Neighbor Mountain and Jeremys Run Loop

Piney Ridge Trail

To Front Royal

Skyline Drive

Elkwallow Wayside

Elkwallow Gap

Elkwallow Picnic Ground

Knob Mountain Cutoff Trail

SHENANDOAH NATIONAL PARK

N

To Thornton Gap

Skyline Drive

Jeremys Run Overlook

Neighbor Mountain Parking Area

P

Blue Ridge

Jeremys Run

Jeremys Run Trail

Knob Mountain Trail

Knob Mountain

Neighbor Mountain Trail

1.5 miles

1.0

1.5 kilometers

0.5

1.0

0

0.5

0

Neighbor Mountain

Moody Creek

Beahm Lane

Jeremys Run

Vaughn Summit Road

Neighbor Mountain and Jeremys Run Loop

In-shape hikers can complete this long loop in a day, but it makes an even better overnight backpack excursion. I have done it both ways. The circuit leaves Elkwallow Picnic Ground (which has water, restrooms, and shaded tables), then heads south-bound on the Appalachian Trail (AT), traversing a pleasant stretch of the world's most famous path-way. Delve into solitude immediately upon joining the Neighbor Mountain Trail, and grab some views on your way to Jeremys Run, one of the prettiest and most productive trout streams in the park. Crisscross to the upper valley of Jeremys Run, then make a final climb, returning to the trailhead.

Best Time

From late spring through midfall, you can make the 15 crossings of Jeremys Run most safely and warmly. The stream will be lower then. Summer is great for fishing and swimming.

Finding the Trail

From Thornton Gap, take Skyline Drive north for 7.4 miles to Elkwallow Picnic Ground at milepost 24.1. Drive to the low end of the picnic area and park. The spur trail to the AT leaves here. The Elkwallow Wayside, a short distance north on Skyline Drive, sells camping supplies, along with food during the warm season in case you don't feel like picnicking.

TRAIL USE
Day Hiking,
Backpacking
LENGTH
14.0 miles,
8.5–10 hours
VERTICAL FEET
±1,650'
DIFFICULTY
– 1 2 3 4 **5** +
TRAIL TYPE
Loop
START & FINISH
N38° 44.457'
W78° 18.715'

FEATURES
Summit
Ridgeline
Stream
Waterfall
Autumn Colors
Wildflowers
Great Views
Swimming
Secluded
Steep

FACILITIES
Camp store (in season)
Picnic area with water
and restrooms

Trail Description

Start your loop on the spur trail leaving Elkwallow Picnic Ground to immediately intersect the AT. ►1 Veer left, heading downhill, southbound through woods. Pass a spur trail on your left to a cool spring just before meeting the Jeremys Run Trail at 0.2 mile. ►2 Make a left here, staying with the AT. Step over the outflow of the spring you just crossed. Begin a mile-long gentle ascent. At 0.7 mile the trail curves around a point and then enters laurel–oak woods atop the ridgeline. Views of Knob Mountain open to your right. Enjoy a forest cruise on a grass-lined, singletrack ribbon in oak and hickory. The broken canopy presents obscured looks into the adjacent valleys and ridges. Begin a mild descent at 2.0 miles. At 2.4 miles, the Thornton River Trail leaves left. ►3 Continue the downgrade, cutting through brushy trees just below Jeremys Run Overlook at 3.1 miles. ►4 There is no trail access to the Skyline Drive viewpoint. Bottom out at 3.1 miles, then resume an uptick, meeting a spur trail left to Skyline Drive at 3.6 miles. ►5

Ridgeline ▲

Autumn Colors 🍁

Begin a winding climb up the western side of Neighbor Mountain, meeting the Neighbor Mountain Trail at 3.9 miles. ►6 Turn right, joining the well-maintained but faint-floored Neighbor Mountain Trail. Expect solitude between here and

Neighbor Mountain and Jeremys Run Loop Elevation Profile

Jeremys Run. The slender, grassy ribbon meanders westerly beneath thick woodland that hosts a dense understory of mountain laurel and smaller trees. The woods become even more attractive and open with oaks and pine above and grass below. The ridgeline slopes sharply off both sides.

 Ridgeline

Hike over a knob to reach a conspicuous rock outcrop on your right at mile 4.9. Several dark rocks stand upright amid smaller rounded boulders. Hop up on a boulder and look over the Shenandoah Valley, which spreads to your right, and the mountains of the park's Central District, which hover on the skyline to your left. Someone must have imagined these upthrust rocks as militaries, for they are known as gendarmes, after the armed French police officers charged with maintaining order.

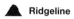 Great Views

Ahead, admire the man-made stonework on and astride the trail. Top out on Neighbor Mountain at 5.7 miles, marked with a concrete post. ▶7 The Potomac Appalachian Trail Club map states the viewless peak, cloaked in brushy, vine-covered woods, to be 2,725 feet. Leave the mountain crest, northwest, descending the steep north slope of The Neighbor. You are in the process of dropping nearly 1,700 feet in 2.6 miles. Be glad you aren't going the other way!

 Summit

 Steep

The foot-pounding drop is moderated with switchbacks. Views between scraggly pines and low-growing blueberries open when the trail is on the ridge's south or west side. You are looking at the Three Sisters, a triple-knobbed ridge to the southwest, and the Shenandoah Valley beyond. The north side of Neighbor Mountain is more deeply wooded and sans vistas. At 7.4 miles, the trail dips to a hollow and briefly joins an old road beside a rocky streambed. ▶8 Reenter pine–oak woods, and resume switchbacking toward the valley floor. Eventually the rapids of Jeremys Run become audible, and the forest correspondingly thickens. Make the last

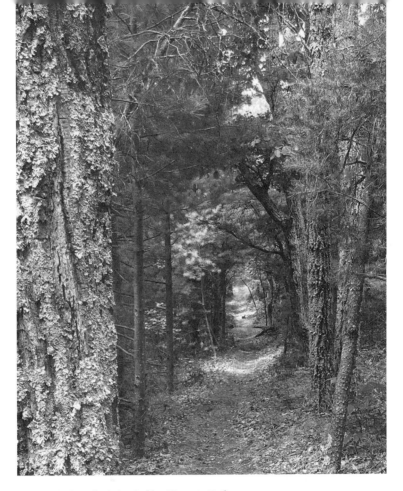

Oaks and pines *flank the Neighbor Mountain Trail.*

Stream

switchback among lush, shaded ferns before meeting the Jeremys Run Trail at 8.3 miles. ▶9 If you want to explore a bit, walk left, downstream, down the Jeremy Run Trail. Some marvelous deep pools form below rock slab cascades. These swimming and fishing holes also sport big sunning rocks.

Swimming

To continue on the loop hike, turn right onto Jeremys Run Trail. Make your first stream crossing, then come to a two-tier waterfall and swimming hole at 9.0 miles. ▶10 Rock walls line the path through here, and white pines rise over former trailside fields.

Sycamores shade the stream where brook trout gather in deep pools. Where rock bluffs crowd Jeremys Run, the path crosses to the other side toward flatter terrain. This pattern of crowding and crossing continues up the valley. Most of the 15 crossings are in the upper valley. In times of high water these fords are dangerous, but most of the time you can cross the run dry-shod.

A steadier grade brings you to the upper valley and the junction with Knob Mountain Cutoff Trail at 13.0 miles. ▶11 Stay right with the Jeremys Run Trail. Wind your way uphill to meet the AT at 13.8 miles. ▶12 From here, backtrack to Elkwallow Picnic Ground, completing the hike at 14.0 miles. ▶13

🚶		MILESTONES
▶1	0.0	Elkwallow Picnic Ground at milepost 24.1
▶2	0.2	Left on AT where Jeremys Run Trail leaves right
▶3	2.4	Thornton River Trail leaves left
▶4	3.1	Pass below Jeremys Run Overlook
▶5	3.6	Spur to Skyline Drive
▶6	3.9	Right on Neighbor Mountain Trail
▶7	5.7	Neighbor Mountain summit
▶8	7.4	Briefly join a roadbed along streambed
▶9	8.3	Right on Jeremys Run Trail
▶10	9.0	Waterfall and swimming hole on right
▶11	13.0	Right on Jeremys Run Trail where Knob Mountain Cutoff Trail leaves left
▶12	13.8	Rejoin the AT
▶13	14.0	Elkwallow Picnic Ground at milepost 24.1

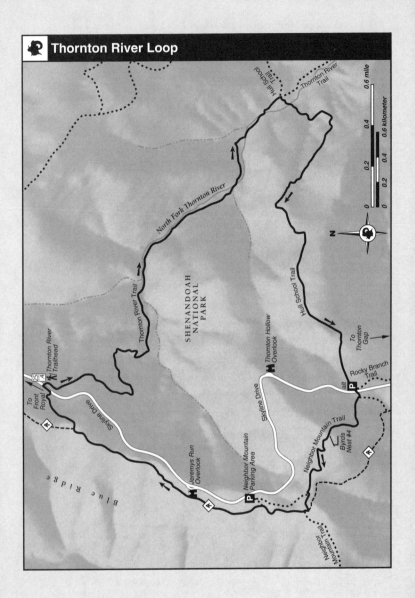

Thornton River Loop

Thornton River Loop

This loop is a quiet hike through history, combined with a little high-country trekking. Leave Skyline Drive to walk the once-settled Thornton Hollow. Here, relics of settlers are scattered onto the landscape. Walk along the alluring North Fork Thornton River, one of the park's more productive trout streams. Wander richly forested flats between creek crossings. Leave the lowlands on the Hull School Trail, angling up a once-settled slope.

The path then crosses Skyline Drive and climbs a peak, where a day-use shelter stands. From here, descend to meet the Appalachian Trail (AT). Trace the AT northbound on a pleasant stretch of path back to the trailhead. I have backpacked this loop on a summer Saturday and not seen a soul. Mine was the only car in the lot too.

Best Time

Spring is a great time to view the wildflowers and see old-home sites before the leaves grow back on the trees. Summer can be good for fishing and backpacking. The lesser-used loop offers decent solitude when other circuits may be busy. Late fall—when the leaves are off and the stream dead-low—is also a good time.

Finding the Trail

Park in the area on the east side of Skyline Drive at milepost 25.4. The Thornton River Trail starts on the left side of the parking area.

TRAIL USE
Day Hiking,
Backpacking
LENGTH
7.9 miles, 4.5–5.5 hours
VERTICAL FEET
±1,500'
DIFFICULTY
– 1 2 3 **4** 5 +
TRAIL TYPE
Loop
START & FINISH
N38° 43.435'
W78° 19.205'

FEATURES
Summit
Ridgeline
Stream
Waterfall
Autumn Colors
Wildflowers
Wildlife
Secluded
Historical Interest

FACILITIES
None

Trail Description

Start your hike by descending from the parking area through a rocky oak–pine–maple–hickory forest on the Thornton Hollow Trail. ▶1 Trace an old settler roadbed on a blue-blazed track. Shortly step over a spring branch. It isn't long before you see the first rock pile, made by farmers clearing stony fields. Curve back north at 0.4 mile, still descending. White oaks and tulip trees are plentiful. The moderate slope made it easy for settlers to use this upper valley for pasture, even for growing corn.

At 0.9 mile, pass near an edifice-like rock pile. This square stone mound was added to year after year, in an attempt to clear what is now forested ground. Curve downhill to cross a tributary of the North Fork Thornton River at 1.0 mile. Rock walls line the settler-road-turned-trail. But it wasn't just wagons and horses rumbling down this track—at 1.1 miles you can see the stripped remnants of an old jalopy. ▶2

Begin paralleling the branch, crossing it a second time. Sycamores, tulip trees, and other hardwoods rise over the waterway, along with white pines. Spicebush and stinging nettle share the understory. Come alongside the North Fork Thornton River. Flats widen on either side of the waterway.

Stream

Historical Interest

Autumn Colors

Thornton River Loop Elevation Profile

Continue down Thornton Hollow. At 1.9 miles, the river squeezes through a rock chute to your left in louder cascades and deeper pools. At 2.2 miles, a thickly wooded flat separates you from the river. Step over a stony tributary that may or may not be flowing. Cross the river at 2.3 miles. The North Fork Thornton River has a highly variable water flow, often braiding when high, but it should be fairly easy to cross except after storms. It is also one of Shenandoah's more productive brook trout streams.

At 2.6 miles, come alongside yet another rock wall. Pass over the outflow of the homesite spring. Just ahead, cross the river again. You are on the right-hand bank. Here, the valley widens. The imprint of humans is visible on both sides of the river. Look for roads, rock walls, and rusty artifacts. Remember, these are cultural resources of the park and should be left where they lay for others to enjoy. Keep down the hollow, and cross the river again at 2.8 miles. Enter a closing field to intersect the Hull School Trail at 2.9 miles. ▶3 The Hull School once stood to the right of you as you face downriver.

Join the Hull School Trail, leading right to cross the watercourse at an island. Here, the trail jumps off and on old settler roads, evidenced by rutted beds and rock walls. Head uphill through straight-trunked cove hardwoods towering over a rock floor. Steepen at a pair of switchbacks, then step over a spring branch at 3.7 miles. This spring likely watered a homesite hereabouts. Continue up, heading off and on old roadbeds amid occasional flats. At 5.0 miles, the trail tops out. You are clearly on an old road, passing through farmland, despite being 2,300 feet in elevation and adjacent to the crest of the Blue Ridge.

Emerge onto Skyline Drive at 5.3 miles. ▶4 Here, the Rocky Branch Trail leaves left. This hike crosses Skyline Drive and heads up a gated fire road marking the beginning of the Neighbor Mountain

 Waterfall

View relics of Shenandoah's pre-park residents on this hike.

Byrds Nest Shelter #4, *atop a knob, proves an irresistible break spot.*

Summit ▲ Trail. Trace this doubletrack trail uphill past a clearing, then make a solid ascent to top out at Byrds Nest Shelter #4 at 5.6 miles. ▶5 This three-sided stone refuge looks east over a grassy clearing. Despite having a fireplace, it is for day use only.

Ridgeline ▲ From here, the yellow-blazed Neighbor Mountain Trail morphs into a singletrack path and drops westerly into pine, oak, and laurel woods. Reach a trail junction at 6.0 miles. Here a spur trail leads right to the Neighbor Mountain Parking Area on Skyline Drive. Keep straight on the Neighbor Mountain Trail to meet the AT at 6.1 miles. ▶6 The hike turns right, northbound, on the heavily trod track. Soon pass another spur to Skyline Drive. Stay with the AT.

Bisect the brush below Jeremys Run Overlook at 6.9 miles. The AT makes for an easy, gently undulating walk under oaks. Meet the upper end of the Thornton River Trail at 7.6 miles. ►7 Turn right, dropping off the ridgeline. One final switchback drops you off just south of the Thornton River Parking Area, and you complete the loop hike at 7.9 miles. ►8

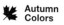 **Autumn Colors**

		MILESTONES
► 1	0.0	Thornton River Parking Area at milepost 25.4
► 2	1.1	Old jalopy to the left of trail
► 3	2.9	Right on Hull School Trail
► 4	5.3	Cross Skyline Drive
► 5	5.6	Byrds Nest Shelter #4
► 6	6.1	Right on the AT
► 7	7.6	Right on Thornton River Trail
► 8	7.9	Thornton River Parking Area at milepost 25.4

Central District

Central District

The Central District is the park's largest ranger district. Not surprisingly, it offers the most hiking opportunities, as well as other park possibilities, ranging from lodging to car camping to guided horseback riding and general visitor services. The Central District, quite wide in sections, begins at Thornton Gap in the north, with east–west US 211 bisecting the park while linking Sperryville and Luray. Skyline Drive runs for 34 miles through the district and accesses the area's major natural features, trailheads, campgrounds, and visitor facilities.

Heading south from Thornton Gap, you will first come to Hazel Country, a sizable trail network that uses old pioneer paths and roads. Hikers will find pioneer evidence in the hills and hollows of the Hazel River and Hughes River Valleys. Loop hikes explore this land of the Old Dominion pioneer, as well as natural features such as Hazel Falls and Cave. Wonderful high-country hikes traverse the spine of the Blue Ridge, including the stellar view from Marys Rock, a must-visit destination. You will run into the first major visitor facility at Skyland, lodging quarters that predate the park's establishment. The shoulder of epic Stony Man Mountain, site of Skyland, is laced with exciting trails. Visit the open outcrops of Stony Man, with its wide panoramas.

And then there's Old Rag. The deservedly popular peak is Virginia's contribution to great mountains of the world. The rock scramble up there is a thrilling challenge, and the views are simply spectacular. Robertson Mountain, Old Rag's neighbor, sports some fair vistas itself and is a destination solitude-seekers will better enjoy. Whiteoak Canyon is one of Shenandoah's most rugged gorges. Through it spills no less than seven major named waterfalls, along with innumerable lesser cataracts that together add up to one whitewater-filled valley. Whiteoak Canyon can be accessed from high and low. A parade of visitors reflects its convenient dual admission. The canyon of Cedar Run, just south of Whiteoak Canyon, is

Opposite and overleaf: *The sharp cliff of Hawksbill (Trail 23, page 159) presents stellar views.*

arguably even rougher. A stony-to-the-extreme trail leads hikers to more waterfalls and swimming holes. It's very popular too.

Hawksbill, the park's highest peak at 4,050 feet, adds to the concentration of notable Central District hiking destinations. It's a fairly easy trek to this crested pinnacle, where a stony brow allows for sweeping views in all directions. Conveniently, an inlaid compass identifies adjacent mountains visible from the top of Hawksbill. Nearby, the Rose River Loop visits a pair of worthy waterfalls and an old mine.

Big Meadows, a highland pasture, offers camping, a lodge, camp store, and visitor center where you can learn more about the park, purchase memorabilia, and participate in ranger programs. Stop by the visitor center when hiking to the vista at Blackrock Mountain and Lewis Falls, one of the park's highest-elevation cataracts. Human history stands prominent again along Mill Prong, where President Herbert Hoover had his retreat, Rapidan Camp. You can tour this preserved aggregation of buildings along with natural features, such as Big Rock Falls and Hazeltop, one of the few areas in the park where rare spruce and fir trees cling to the heights.

Hikers can use trails that link Shenandoah National Park with the state-owned lands of Rapidan Wildlife Management Area. Travel along the waterfall- and trout-rich Staunton River on your way to Bear Church Rock, a secluded vista with one of the greatest names in the entire Appalachian chain. Another hike heads deep down the Conway River Valley, a big and brawling stream. Or tackle the Bearfence Mountain Rock Scramble, a view-laden adventure through a boulder garden. Lewis Mountain, with its campground, cabins, and fine picnic area, offers a tamer experience.

Things quiet down near Pocosin Mission, a short walk from Skyline Drive. Visit the ruins of a Christian ministry from pre-park days. Hikers often incorporate a meal into their hike at rustic South River Picnic Ground. One walk leads to South River Falls, a cataract you can enjoy from above and below. Wildflowers carpet this valley in spring. US 33, which connects Elkton in the west to Stanardsville in the east, marks the southern boundary of the Central District.

Permits

Permits are not required for day hiking. Backpackers must get a permit to stay in the backcountry. Simple self-registration stations are located at Thornton Gap Entrance Station, Big Meadows Visitor Center, and Swift Run Gap Entrance Station on Skyline Drive, and at Old Rag Fee Station on the park's east side.

Central District

Middle
Mountain

Shenandoah River

340

Luray

211

211

340B

340B

689

611

Hershberger
Hill

Three
Sisters

211

Pine
Mountain

Marys
Rock

Thornton Gap
Entrance
Station

Oventop
Mountain

To
Sperryville

211

14

15 16

Redmans
Mountain

231

17

Bushtop

18

19 20 21

Hawksbill

23

22

Old Rag
Mountain

Etlan

Devils
Tanyard

24

25

Big Meadows
Visitor Center

SHENANDOAH
NATIONAL
PARK

26

Dulaney
Mountain

Mitchells
Mountain

231

Grindstone
Mountain

Hazeltop

27 29 30

Fork
Mountain

Carpenter
Mountain

Skyline Drive

31

Lewis
Mountain

Sag Top

28

Utz
Hightop

Dean
Mountain

32

Kirtley
Mountain

Yager
Mountain

231

Madison

33

Swift Run Gap
Entrance
Station

To
Elkton

To
Gordonsville

N

33

0   1   2   3 miles

0 1 2   3 kilometers

28

Ferns *at Stony Man Loop (Trail 19, page 137)*

Maps

For the Central District, here are the relevant U.S. Geological Survey 7.5-minute (1:24,000-scale) topographic quadrangles, listed in geographic order as you hike along your route:

Trail 14: *Old Rag Mountain* and *Thornton Gap*
Trail 15: *Thornton Gap*
Trail 16: *Thornton Gap* and *Old Rag Mountain*
Trail 17: *Old Rag Mountain*
Trail 18: *Old Rag Mountain*
Trail 19: *Big Meadows* and *Old Rag Mountain*
Trail 20: *Big Meadows* and *Old Rag Mountain*
Trail 21: *Old Rag Mountain*
Trail 22: *Big Meadows* and *Old Rag Mountain*
Trail 23: *Big Meadows*
Trail 24: *Big Meadows*
Trail 25: *Big Meadows*
Trail 26: *Big Meadows* and *Fletcher*
Trail 27: *Madison, Fletcher,* and *Big Meadows*
Trail 28: *Madison* and *Fletcher*
Trail 29: *Fletcher*
Trail 30: *Fletcher*
Trail 31: *Fletcher*
Trail 32: *Fletcher*
Trail 33: *Elkton East* and *Fletcher*

Central District

TRAIL	Difficulty	Length	Type	USES & ACCESS	TERRAIN	NATURE	OTHER
14	3	7.2	Out-and-Back	Day Hiking	Ridgeline	Autumn Colors	Great Views, Geological Interest
15	3	5.2	Out-and-Back	Day Hiking, Child-Friendly	Ridgeline, Stream, Waterfall	Autumn Colors, Wildflowers	Geological Interest
16	5	16.8	Loop	Day Hiking, Backpacking	Ridgeline, Stream, Waterfall	Autumn Colors, Wildflowers	Great Views, Secluded, Historical Interest, Geological Interest
17	3	2.8	Out-and-Back	Day Hiking	Ridgeline, Stream	Autumn Colors, Wildflowers	Historical Interest
18	5	9.1	Loop	Day Hiking, Pets Prohibited	Summit, Ridgeline, Stream	Autumn Colors, Wildflowers	Great Views, Geological Interest
19	3	3.4	Loop	Day Hiking, Pets Prohibited	Summit, Ridgeline	Autumn Colors, Wildflowers	Great Views, Historical Interest, Geological Interest
20	4	6.8	Out-and-Back	Day Hiking	Summit, Ridgeline, Stream	Autumn Colors	Great Views
21	4	5.2	Out-and-Back	Day Hiking	Stream, Waterfall	Wildflowers	Great Views, Steep, Geological Interest
22	4	3.4	Out-and-Back	Day Hiking	Stream, Waterfall	Autumn Colors	Steep, Geological Interest
23	2	2.2	Out-and-Back	Day Hiking	Summit	Autumn Colors	Great Views
24	3	4.0	Loop	Day Hiking, Backpacking	Stream, Waterfall	Autumn Colors, Wildflowers	Historical Interest, Geological Interest
25	3	3.3	Loop	Day Hiking, Backpacking	Summit, Ridgeline, Stream, Waterfall	Autumn Colors, Wildflowers	Great Views, Geological Interest
26	4	7.2	Loop	Day Hiking, Backpacking	Summit, Ridgeline, Stream, Waterfall	Autumn Colors, Wildflowers, Wildlife	Great Views, Historical Interest
27	5	18.6	Loop	Day Hiking, Backpacking	Ridgeline, Stream, Waterfall	Autumn Colors	Great Views, Camping, Swimming, Secluded, Historical Interest, Geological Interest
28	5	7.6	Out-and-Back	Day Hiking, Backpacking	Summit, Stream, Waterfall	Autumn Colors	Great Views, Swimming, Secluded, Historical Interest, Geological Interest
29	4	9.4	Out-and-Back	Day Hiking	Ridgeline	Autumn Colors	Great Views, Secluded
30	5	12.0	Loop	Day Hiking, Backpacking, Pets Prohibited	Ridgeline, Stream, Waterfall	Autumn Colors, Wildflowers, Old-Growth Forest	Great Views, Historical Interest, Geological Interest
31	3	1.1	Loop	Day Hiking, Pets Prohibited	Ridgeline	Autumn Colors	Great Views, Geological Interest
32	2	2.0	Out-and-Back	Day Hiking, Child-Friendly	Ridgeline	Autumn Colors, Wildflowers, Old-Growth Forest	Great Views, Historical Interest
33	3	4.5	Loop	Day Hiking	Stream, Waterfall	Autumn Colors, Wildflowers	Geological Interest

Legend

TYPE
- Loop
- Out-and-Back

DIFFICULTY
- 1 2 3 4 5 +
- less   more

USES & ACCESS
- Day Hiking
- Backpacking
- Child-Friendly
- Pets Prohibited

TERRAIN
- Summit
- Ridgeline
- Stream
- Waterfall

NATURE
- Autumn Colors
- Wildflowers
- Wildlife
- Old-Growth Forest

FEATURES
- Great Views
- Camping
- Swimming
- Secluded
- Steep
- Historical Interest
- Geological Interest

Central District

Old Rag Loop 131

This well-loved Shenandoah classic is the most difficult hike in this entire guidebook. Strike up the north slope of Old Rag, emerging onto a massive granite slab, revealing incredible panoramas. Enter a maze of boulders, with some bona fide rock scrambling to reach the summit with stellar views. Leave the rugged mountaintop, and reenter the lowlands via the pretty valley of Brokenback Run on a foot-relieving gravel fire road.

TRAIL 18

Day Hiking,
Pets Prohibited
9.1 miles, Loop
Difficulty: 1 2 3 4 **5**

Stony Man Loop 137

Hike to the summit of Stony Man Mountain, where cliffs rise 3,000 feet above the Shenandoah Valley and present superlative panoramas. Take the Little Stony Man Trail to Little Stony Man, where more overlooks await. Return along the Passamaquoddy Trail, where still more views can be seen. Stop by Furnace Spring, once used in a copper-mining operation, before completing this highlight-laden loop.

TRAIL 19

Day Hiking,
Pets Prohibited
3.4 miles, Loop
Difficulty: 1 2 **3** 4 5

Robertson Mountain 143

Before reaching this lesser-visited peak, explore a highland cove and wetland on the all-access Limberlost Trail. Join Old Rag Fire Road, where the walking is easy. A more traditional singletrack foot trail takes you the last mile to the outcrops of Robertson Mountain. At the summit, various rocky points avail sweeping views in three directions.

TRAIL 20

Day Hiking
6.8 miles, Out-and-back
Difficulty: 1 2 3 **4** 5

Falls of Whiteoak Canyon. 149

Explore six sequentially numbered falls while ascending a rugged gorge with everywhere-you-look beauty. Top out on a rock promontory with a view of the uppermost falls. Beware the crowds during nice weather.

TRAIL 21

Day Hiking
5.2 miles, Out-and-back
Difficulty: 1 2 3 **4** 5

Hazeltop and Rapidan Camp Loop . . .175

This loop leads over Hazeltop, third-highest peak in the park, and then traces attractive Laurel Prong Trail down to Rapidan Camp, President Herbert Hoover's woodland getaway. There's much to see at the camp; you can even embark on a self-guided interpretive tour. Return to Milam Gap via Mill Prong Trail, and view Big Rock Falls along the way.

TRAIL 26

Day Hiking,
Backpacking
7.2 miles, Loop
Difficulty: 1 2 3 **4** 5

Staunton River Loop. 181

This circuit travels high and low, sporting mountaintop vistas as well as park history. However, most of the adventure is along the Staunton River and its mother stream, the Rapidan River. Both waterways deliver national park–level scenery, including waterfalls and big pools.

TRAIL 27

Day Hiking,
Backpacking
18.6 miles, Loop
Difficulty: 1 2 3 4 **5**

Bear Church Rock via Staunton River. 187

Hike up the Staunton River Valley, a classic mountain vale centered with a pool-and-chute trout stream. Wind into the high country, and emerge at a rock promontory that offers both solitude and first-rate views.

TRAIL 28

Day Hiking,
Backpacking
7.6 miles, Out-and-back
Difficulty: 1 2 3 4 **5**

Bear Church Rock from Bootens Gap. 193

This solitude-laden high-country hike leads along the ridge of Jones Mountain to a fine view. The hiking along Jones Mountain is some of Shenandoah's finest. Stay above 3,000 feet on trail that is never steep for long and mostly level, making it a glorious 9 mountain miles.

TRAIL 29

Day Hiking
9.4 miles, Out-and-back
Difficulty: 1 2 3 **4** 5

TRAIL 30

Day Hiking,
Backpacking,
Pets Prohibited
12.0 miles, Loop
Difficulty: 1 2 3 4 **5**

Conway River Loop. 197

Leave the Blue Ridge, and follow the scenic Conway
River through an archetypal Appalachian valley.
Next, head into the high country on the seldom-
trampled Slaughter Trail, passing pioneer homesites.
Complete your trip by clambering over Bearfence
Mountain, with its 360-degree views, on a short but
challenging rock scramble.

TRAIL 31

Day Hiking,
Pets Prohibited
1.1 miles, Loop
Difficulty: 1 2 **3** 4 5

Bearfence Mountain Rock Scramble. .205

Reward yourself with 360-degree views from open
outcrops along the well-marked trail that combines
with the Appalachian Trail to make a short but
exhilarating loop. The trek does require the use of
hands and feet in a few places, but it is neither dangerous nor difficult and can be done by all but the
youngest and oldest of Shenandoah trail trekkers.

TRAIL 32

Day Hiking,
Child-Friendly
2.0 miles, Out-and-back
Difficulty: 1 **2** 3 4 5

Pocosin Mission 209

Take a short walk into the past. The wide and easy
Pocosin Fire Road heads to ruins of the Pocosin
Mission. Explore the ruins of the mission and other
nearby signs of habitation on a child-friendly trek.

TRAIL 33

Day Hiking
4.5 miles, Loop
Difficulty: 1 2 **3** 4 5

South River Falls Loop 213

Make an easy descent to see South River Falls drop
80 feet over a rock face from a perched vista. Go farther to the base of the falls in a rich spring-wildflower
zone. Climb from the South River watershed back to
the former mountaintop pastureland. The falls are
worth the exercise.

Marys Rock via The Pinnacle

The hike over The Pinnacle to Marys Rock traverses the most spectacular section of the Appalachian Trail (AT) through Shenandoah National Park. The views are expansive and frequent. And hiking to a view is always more rewarding than driving to a view. Panoramas open up shortly after you leave Pinnacles Picnic Ground. A climb leads you to The Pinnacle, which has an outstanding vista. Still more views await before what many Shenandoah old-timers feel is the best vista in the entire park—Marys Rock. This hike's rewards far outstrip the effort it requires. Its elevation changes only amount to climbs and drops of 450 feet each—not bad for this park, not bad at all.

TRAIL USE
Day Hiking

LENGTH
7.2 miles, 4–5 hours

VERTICAL FEET
±450'

DIFFICULTY
– 1 2 **3** 4 5 +

TRAIL TYPE
Out-and-back

START & FINISH
N38° 37.483'
W78° 20.539'

FEATURES
Ridgeline
Autumn Colors
Great Views
Geological Interest

FACILITIES
Picnic tables
Restrooms
Water

Best Time

Fall through spring is the best period for maximizing the multiple stunning views along this ridgeline. The weather is mild even in summer, since the trail never dips below 3,200 feet.

Finding the Trail

The Pinnacles Picnic Ground is located at milepost 36.7 on Skyline Drive. From the Thornton Gap Entrance Station, take Skyline Drive south for 5.2 miles to the Pinnacles Picnic Ground entrance. Pick up the AT on your right as you top out in the picnic area, before the road starts looping around. If the picnic area is closed (as it is in winter), simply start at Jewell Hollow Overlook at milepost 36.4. Pick up the AT at the south end of the overlook.

Marys Rock via The Pinnacle

Skyline Drive

Thornton Gap

211

211

To
Luray

SHENANDOAH
NATIONAL
PARK

Marys
Rock

669

(no access)

tunnel

Tunnel Parking
Overlook

Buck Hollow
Overlook

Hazel Mountain
Overlook

Buck Hollow Trail

Blue Ridge

Meadow Spring Trail

Skyline Drive

Byrds
Nest #3

Leading Ridge Trail

Jewell
Hollow
Overlook

The
Pinnacle

Pinnacles
Picnic
Ground

36
7

Skyline Drive

To
Swift Run
Gap

Pinnacle
Overlook

Hannah Run Trail

N

0   0.2   0.4   0.6 mile

0   0.2   0.4   0.6 kilometer

Trail Description

Pick up the AT in the grassy margin to the right of the picnic area entrance road. ▶1 Head right, northbound, for Jewell Hollow Overlook. Pass some spruce trees that were likely planted. Views immediately open to your left as you travel along a stony upthrust escarpment. Dip to reach the Jewell Hollow Overlook at 0.2 mile. ▶2 The AT goes south a short distance before making a switchback to head north. Come to a small field below the overlook. Enjoy an unobstructed opening to the west. Lake Arrowhead lies below. Begin to climb beyond the field. Reenter woodland, coming to a trail junction at 0.5 mile. ▶3 Pass the Leading Ridge Trail, and continue north on the AT.

The path tunnels through an understory of mountain laurel in dense woodland. At 0.9 mile enter a forest area littered with massive gray boulders. The trees are short because of thin soils and rough climatic conditions atop the mountains. Meander amid the boulders, watching for unusual stacked stones that seem likely to fall. Open onto The Pinnacle (3,730') at mile 1.2. ▶4 The rock outcrop has a sheer drop-off. Be prepared for an incredible view of Virginia mountains and valleys to the west. You can see Luray below and on a clear day look north at the balance of the park, including your destination—Marys Rock, a mere bump along the ridge from here. Be careful on these jagged, uneven rocks.

The AT continues north and descends a series of switchbacks in very stony woods. Slip over to the southeast side of the mountain. In a gap, reach the Byrds Nest Shelter #3 at 2.1 miles. ▶5 The three-sided camping structure is open to AT thru-hikers, defined as three consecutive nights or longer on the AT. This stone shelter has a picnic table and provides a respite from the elements, but don't expect the water fountain to work. A privy stands just

From this trail, soak in what is arguably the best panorama in the park.

 Great Views

 Autumn Colors

Geological Interest

 Great Views

The Pinnacle *offers northward views of the Blue Ridge and the North District of the park beyond.*

ahead. Follow the service road that leads from the shelter to Skyline Drive for a short distance. Veer left at the intersection, staying on the AT. The service road drops right to a spring and Skyline Drive.

Another westward view opens at mile 2.5, soon after a switchback to the left. You can also look back at The Pinnacle and its outcrops. A grassy flat here beckons a rest. Ahead, a rock promontory offers more looks at 2.7 miles, including Stony Man

Marys Rock via The Pinnacle Elevation Profile

Mountain. The Meadow Spring Trail leaves right at mile 2.9. ►6 Begin climbing for a quarter mile. The trail levels as it approaches the backside of Marys Rock. Continue downhill to the Marys Rock spur trail at 3.5 miles. ►7 Turn left on the spur trail and rise to Marys Rock, reaching it at 3.6 miles. ►8

 Great Views

The panorama from the huge outcrop ranges far and wide. Choose your viewing spot. To the north, easy views of many Blue Ridge peaks open. The town of Luray and the Shenandoah Valley are visible to the west. The Thornton Gap Entrance Station stands clearly below. Please respect closures and sensitive vegetation in this area. Decide for yourself if Marys Rock has the best view in the park. Just be careful doing it. It is undeniably one of Shenandoah's best scenic spots, and a personal favorite of mine.

Great Views

↟	**MILESTONES**	
►1	0.0	Pinnacles Picnic Ground
►2	0.2	Jewell Hollow Overlook
►3	0.5	Leading Ridge Trail leads left
►4	1.2	Vista from The Pinnacle
►5	2.1	Byrds Nest Shelter #3
►6	2.9	Meadow Spring Trail leaves right
►7	3.5	Spur trail to Marys Rock
►8	3.6	Marys Rock

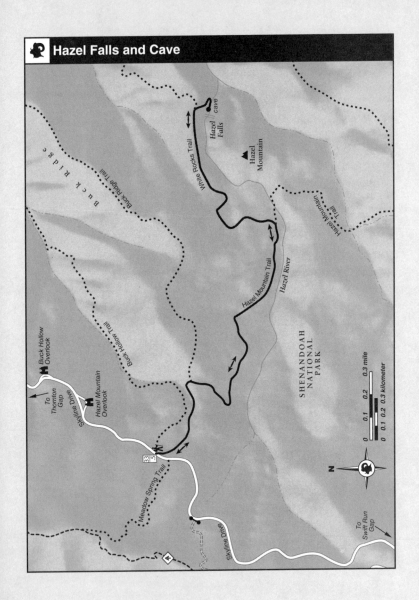

Hazel Falls and Cave

Hazel Falls

Hazel cave

Hazel Mountain

White Rocks Trail

Buck Ridge

Buck Ridge Trail

Hazel Mountain Trail

Hazel River

Hazel Mountain Trail

SHENANDOAH NATIONAL PARK

Buck Hollow Overlook

Buck Hollow Trail

To Thornton Gap

Skyline Drive

Hazel Mountain Overlook

Meadow Spring Trail

Skyline Drive

To Swift Run Gap

0   0.1   0.2   0.3 mile
0   0.1 0.2 0.3 kilometer

N

Hazel Falls and Cave

This hike takes you into "Hazel Country," a heavily settled area in pre-park days. The route traverses hill and hollow for the Hazel River, where a rock indentation forms a natural shelter beside a waterfall, all within a deep stone cathedral. All in all, it's a good destination. The difficulty of this hike is hard to rate: the first 2.4-mile portion is a moderate stroll on old settler roads, but the last 0.3-mile trek to the cave and falls is on a steep, rough footpath. Though rugged, this section is short; all but small children should make it.

Best Time

The falls flow more during winter and spring. On summer weekends fellow hikers head to the glen where the falls and cave are enclosed. Winter offers solitude aplenty and an iced-over cataract.

Finding the Trail

The trailhead is located east of milepost 33.5 of Skyline Drive at Meadow Spring. The parking area is on the east side of Skyline Drive. It is 2 miles south of the Thornton Gap Entrance Station on Skyline Drive.

Trail Description

Leave Skyline Drive on the Hazel Mountain Trail, formerly the Hazel Mountain Fire Road. ►1 Come to a trail junction at 0.4 mile. ►2 Veer right, still on the Hazel Mountain Trail, as the Buck Ridge

TRAIL USE
Day Hiking,
Child-Friendly

LENGTH
5.2 miles, 2.5–3.5 hours

VERTICAL FEET
±950'

DIFFICULTY
– 1 2 **3** 4 5 +

TRAIL TYPE
Out-and-back

START & FINISH
N38° 38.298'
W78° 18.828'

FEATURES
Ridgeline
Stream
Waterfall
Autumn Colors
Wildflowers
Geological Interest

FACILITIES
None

▲ **Ridgeline**

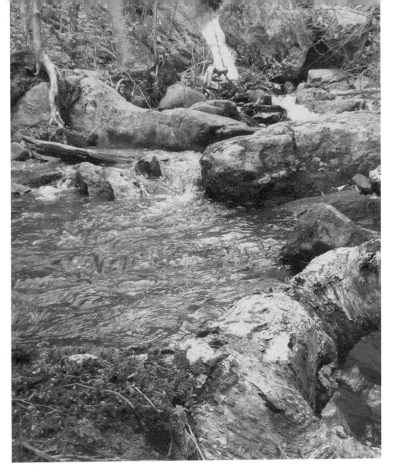

Boulders roil *the waters of the Hazel River.*

Hazel Falls and Cave Elevation Profile

Trail drops left. Striped maples crowd the path and form a dense canopy overhead. Striped maples are a smaller tree, easily recognized by the vertical stripes on green bark and typical maple leaves, albeit larger than red maples. They grow primarily in the Northeast, where they are nicknamed moosewood. Striped maples stretch south along the spine of the Appalachians down to Georgia. "Moosewood" derives from moose feeding on the trees' bark in winter. Deer, beavers, and rabbits also feed on striped maples during the cold season.

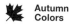 **Autumn Colors**

Soon the trail bears left, levels out, and crosses several small spring branches dribbling down Buck Ridge. The trail sidles alongside the Hazel River at mile 1.0. The valley spreads wide into a cove— farmland way back when. Continue along the river, and turn left on the White Rocks Trail at mile 1.6. ▶3 The path ascends slightly, leaving Hazel River, then levels out along an old road shaded by tulips and maples. Other old roads veer off this trail, but the main path is evident. Large boulders are strewn about the forest, which morphs to pine and chestnut oak as the trail tops out on the ridge. Wild azaleas bloom in May.

 Stream

The trail becomes rockier and descends some-what. A watery symphony drifts from below. Come to a trail junction at mile 2.4. ▶4 The White Rocks Trail continues forward, while the official Cave and Falls Trail footpath veers right (it used to be a user-created manway). Follow the Cave and Falls Trail downhill. The trail then dives down a steep path mitigated by stone steps. Carefully descend to the river. Hazel Mountain rises across the way. River cascades spill down the valley below.

 Wildflowers

Reach the river at 2.5 miles. Notice the peel-ing trunks of the many yellow birches. Turn right, following the footpath upstream. Pass a sizable trailside tulip tree as you dance betwixt boulders. Reach the rock shelter on your right just before the

 Stream

Geological Interest waterfall. A natural rock amphitheater enfolds the scene. The rock indentation lies on your right at the base of a huge, granite bluff—quite a sturdy roof. ►5 The cave is about 10 feet deep, 25 feet wide, and 7 feet high. It gets a little deeper in one spot. Hazel Falls slices about 25 feet down a narrow chute into a deep pool, and is but one piece of this picturesque

Waterfall mountain mosaic.

The rock notch makes this a good rainy-day destination. If you explore the rest of the boulders carefully, you will find more open overhangs, as well as other waterfall observation points. Relax and take it all in.

🚶	**MILESTONES**	
►1	0.0	Meadow Spring Parking Area at milepost 33.5
►2	0.4	Stay right as Buck Ridge Trail leaves left
►3	1.6	Left on White Rocks Trail
►4	2.4	Right on Cave and Falls Trail
►5	2.7	Hazel Falls and Cave

Hazel Country Loop

This big loop—great for backpacking—courses through an interconnected trail network cobbled together from a web of pre-park roads where settlers once lived in highland isolation. You'll find natural highlights such as overlooks and waterfalls, as well as settler history, from chimneys to rock walls to rusted-out washtubs. After visiting Hazel Falls and Cave, you'll enjoy vistas from White Rocks before returning to the Hazel River. A steep climb up Sams Ridge returns you to the upland flats of Hazel Mountain, where the hiking is easy. The catchily named Hot Short Mountain Trail drops you by the Hughes River with its pools and rapids, and then Hannah Run Trail returns you to the highlands.

Best Time

You'll find the myriad pre-park pioneer homesites more easily when the leaves are off. Spring will have wildflowers, and the varied forest will be a cornucopia of color in fall, but stream crossings can be more challenging. Solitude will be found most anytime beyond Hazel Falls and Cave.

Finding the Trail

The trailhead is on the east side of milepost 33.5 of Skyline Drive, Meadow Spring. The parking area is on the east side of Skyline Drive and can be accessed by driving south for 2 miles from the Thornton Gap entrance on Skyline Drive.

TRAIL USE
Day Hiking,
Backpacking
LENGTH
16.8 miles,
8.5–10.5 hours
VERTICAL FEET
±1,600
DIFFICULTY
– 1 2 3 4 **5** +
TRAIL TYPE
Loop
START & FINISH
N38° 38.298'
W78° 18.828'

FEATURES
Ridgeline
Stream
Waterfall
Autumn Colors
Wildflowers
Great Views
Secluded
Steep
Historical Interest
Geological Interest

FACILITIES
None

Hazel Country Loop

Meadow Spring Parking Area

To Thornton Gap

Buck Hollow Trail

Buck Ridge Trail

White Rocks Trail

Hazel River

Hazel Mountain Trail

Hazel Falls

SHENANDOAH NATIONAL PARK

Hazel River Trail

Skyline Drive

Catlett Spur Trail

Hannah Run Trail

Runyon Run

Hazel Mountain Trail

Hazel Mountain

Sams Run

Hazel River Trail

Catlett Mountain Trail

chimney

Catlett Mountain

Hannah Run

Hazel Mountain Trail

Sams Ridge Trail

600

Short Mountain

chimney

Broad Hollow Trail

Pine Hill Gap Trail

681

Hannah Run Trail

Hot Mountain

Nicholson Hollow Trail

Hot Short Mountain Trail

Rocky Run

Nicholson Hollow Trail

N

0   0.3   0.6   0.9 mile

0   0.3   0.6   0.9 kilometer

A rustic trail sign *marks the path.*

Trail Description

The Hazel Mountain Trail takes you away from Skyline Drive ►1 and into Hazel Country, passing the Buck Hollow Trail and Buck Ridge Trail ►2 in the first half mile. At 1.0 mile, you'll come alongside the uppermost Hazel River, more a small creek at this point. Head down the valley at an easy grade, then meet the White Rocks Trail at 1.6 miles. ►3 Turn left on the White Rocks Trail, entering piney woods and running along a ridge.

 Stream

 Ridgeline

At 2.4 miles, ►4 take the spur right for 0.3 mile down to Hazel Falls and Cave on a steep path with elaborate rock work designed to combat erosion. After coming to the Hazel River, turn right upstream under a mantle of imposing bluffs to reach the 25-foot slide falls and the nearby modest cave ►5 at 2.7 miles.

 Waterfall

Backtrack, clambering up to the White Rocks Trail, and turn right, heading east. Find a view ►6 back toward Skyline Drive, Buck Ridge, and Marys Rock at 3.1 miles. Roll over the White Rocks with

 Great Views

more down than up. At 3.6 miles, find an outcrop left of the trail with a view to the Piedmont.

Leave the ridge of White Rocks at 3.8 miles, dropping right from a gap, headlong toward the Hazel River, which you reach at 4.0 miles. ▶7 Rock-hop the stream; then cruise a waterside flat to join the Hazel River Trail at 4.1 miles. Keep downstream, enjoying the woods and waters of the scenic river valley. Four stream crossings keep you hopping over rocks, exploring both banks of the waterway. Enjoy a half mile free of fords, cruising under sycamores. At 5.6 miles, step over Sams Run before turning right onto Sams Ridge Trail. ▶8 The Sams Ridge Trail wastes no time in climbing as you curve out and back into the national park. Keep ascending among oaks and trailside boulders.

At 7.0 miles, level off at an old-home site and spring. Catch your breath on the flattish track before meeting the Broad Hollow Trail at 7.4 miles. ▶9 Turn right here. At 7.6 miles, ▶10 turn left on the Hazel Mountain Trail. Enjoy more easy hiking in uplands to intersect the Catlett Mountain Trail ▶11 at 8.2 miles. Keep straight with the pine-bordered Hazel Mountain Trail.

Trail intersections continue to come fast and frequently. At 8.7 miles, meet the Pine Hill Gap Trail,

Stream

Wildflowers �֎

Steep ⛰

Hazel Country Loop Elevation Profile

but turn right at the intersection, ►12 joining the Hot Short Mountain Trail. Look for views of Old Rag as the path takes you along Catlett Mountain's slope; then aim for the hollow that divides Hot Mountain from Short Mountain. At 9.7 miles, the path leads past a homesite marked by an old chimney. Cross a wide, rocky, and shallow stream, then hike along a bluff edge as the stream you just crossed dives for the lowlands. Enter formerly inhabited flats laced with myriad rock walls then come to the Hughes River and the Nicholson Hollow Trail at 10.8 miles.

The historic circuit turns right, ►13 up the Nicholson Hollow Trail. Step over Hannah Run; then turn right on the Hannah Run Trail at 11.1 miles. ►14 Gently rise into the formerly inhabited vale, looking for pioneer evidence. At 12.6 miles, hike beside another chimney in an unlikely homesite location (very sloped terrain); then descend back to now-small Hannah Run. Make a tough quarter-mile ascent from the stream.

Milder grades lead you to a trail intersection at 13.3 miles. The Hannah Run Trail leaves left—our hike joins the Catlett Mountain Trail right ►15 on a downgrade. At 13.4 miles, reach another intersection. Turn left ►16 on the Catlett Spur Trail, working on and off an old road descending through Runyon Run's upper reaches.

At 14.6 miles, head left ►17 on the Hazel Mountain Trail. Top out on a hill then dip to rock-hop upper Hazel River at 15.1 miles. It's just 0.1 mile farther to the White Rocks Trail; note that you've been here before. From this point, ►18 retrace your steps up the Hazel Mountain Trail, returning to Skyline Drive ►19 at 16.8 miles, completing the historic hike.

Discover Shenandoah's pioneer past.

Stream

Historical Interest

Steep

Autumn Colors

Stream

MILESTONES

▶1	0.0	Meadow Spring Parking Area, milepost 33.5
▶2	0.4	Buck Ridge Trail leaves left
▶3	1.6	Left on White Rocks Trail
▶4	2.4	Spur to Hazel Falls and Cave
▶5	2.7	Hazel Falls and Cave
▶6	3.1	View, another view 0.5 mile ahead
▶7	4.0	Cross Hazel River
▶8	5.6	Right on Sams Ridge Trail
▶9	7.4	Right on Broad Hollow Trail
▶10	7.6	Left on Hazel Mountain Trail
▶11	8.2	Intersect Catlett Mountain Trail
▶12	8.7	Right on Hot Short Mountain Trail
▶13	10.8	Right on Nicholson Hollow Trail
▶14	11.1	Right on Hannah Run Trail
▶15	13.3	Right on Catlett Mountain Trail
▶16	13.4	Left on Catlett Spur Trail
▶17	14.6	Left on Hazel Mountain Trail
▶18	15.2	Meet White Rocks Trail, backtrack left on Hazel Mountain Trail
▶19	16.8	Meadow Spring Parking Area, milepost 33.5

Corbin Cabin Hike

Do you want to visit an intact, authentic Shenandoah pioneer cabin and get a glimpse of settlers' lifeways? And get there using a steep trail created and tramped well before Shenandoah was a national park? If you find the above appealing, here's something to sweeten the pot: Corbin Cabin is available for overnight rental by the public! Even if you don't spend the night, this is still a worthy destination. Not only is the cabin interesting, but the surrounding upper Hughes River is a naturally alluring locale. The brevity of the hike—1.4 miles each way—makes up for the thousand-foot elevation change. If you take your time going up or down, almost anyone can make it.

Best Time

This is a fine year-round destination. No matter what season, visiting the historic Corbin Cabin will give you insight into pre-park pioneer life. Even if the Hughes River is excessively high in spring, you can still see the cabin without having to make the crossing.

Finding the Trail

The Corbin Cabin Cutoff Trail is on the east side of Skyline Drive at milepost 37.9. The parking area has seven spaces and is on the west side of the road. The trailhead is on a hilly curve and is easily missed.

Trail Description

Leave the east side of Skyline Drive on the Corbin Cabin Cutoff Trail. ▶1 This path was not created by park personnel but was simply beaten down by settlers of these Potomac Highlands. The national

TRAIL USE
Day Hiking
LENGTH
2.8 miles, 2.5–3.5 hours
VERTICAL FEET
±1,020'
DIFFICULTY
− 1 2 **3** 4 5 +
TRAIL TYPE
Out-and-back
START & FINISH
N38° 36.938'
W78° 21.052'

FEATURES
Ridgeline
Stream
Autumn Colors
Wildflowers
Historical Interest

FACILITIES
Rental cabin

park generally builds trails with a lesser gradient and takes into account several factors, such as minimizing erosion, stabilizing the trailbed, avoiding sensitive locations for flora and fauna, and routing toward scenic locales. Park personnel have since added waterbars, cleared trees, and strategically placed rocks to keep the trail from washing away.

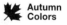
Visit an
intact authentic
pioneer cabin.

Enter hardwoods of birch, striped maple, and oak. Grasses wave across the forest floor. Quickly join a rib ridge emanating from the crest of Shenandoah. Pines and mountain laurel increase in number on this xeric hilltop. Thorofare Mountain rises to your right, as does Stony Man Mountain.

▲ Ridgeline

✸ Autumn Colors

The path steepens at 0.4 mile. It has to lose that elevation sooner or later. At 0.5 mile, the trail turns off the ridge and into a hollow. Reach the head of the hollow at 0.7 mile. ▶2 You are halfway. A trickling branch gurgles amid the rocks, falling to feed the Hughes River. Wildflowers grace the trailside in spring. Lots of rock piles scattered throughout the hollow are signs of cultivation, perhaps by George Corbin himself. Look also for rock walls and overgrown roads. At 1.2 miles, the trail comes alongside a conspicuous rock wall. Step over a little spring branch. The woods are starting to flatten out somewhat. Look right for a narrow path leading uphill to an old pioneer cemetery.

✿ Wildflowers

The Hughes River greets you with a watery song. Look to your right in a flat before the stream to see the remnants of a forgotten structure. Its floor and roof are still intact, but most of the walls have collapsed.

 Stream

Rock-hop the Hughes River. To your left, the Nicholson Hollow Trail has come up 4.0 miles from the community of Nethers. It leads right up to Skyline Drive. The Corbin Cabin stands in front of you, in a small clearing kept open to reduce the possibility of fire taking down the historic structure. ▶3 If it is unoccupied, the building will be closed tightly, but you still can take a seat on the porch to admire the view. The clearing opens to river, rock, and forest, all protected by national park status. Most pioneer cabins were dismantled, but luckily this one was spared for us to experience. It received a restorative makeover in 2017.

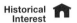
Historical Interest

When George Corbin built his two-story, wood-and-chinking cabin on the banks of the upper Hughes River in 1910, deep in the Potomac Highlands of Virginia, he never imagined it would become a national park attraction on the National Register of Historic Places. Corbin lived in his creation until 1938, when Shenandoah National Park bought him out and he moved outside the newly established boundaries. A legend persists that the cabin is haunted by George's wife Nee who died there during childbirth in the winter of 1924. If you are brave enough to stay, obtain more cabin rental information at patc.net.

🚶 MILESTONES

▶1   0.0   Corbin Cabin Parking Area at milepost 37.9
▶2   0.7   Turn down the hollow toward Hughes River
▶3   1.4   Corbin Cabin

Corbin Cabin Hike Elevation Profile

Old Rag Loop

Old Rag is Shenandoah National Park's addition to the great mountains of America. The granite-topped peak is the park's most recognizable and beloved summit. It is famed for its boulder scramble and the multiplicity of views from the rock protuberances adorning its flanks. And the Old Rag loop is a Shenandoah classic, a must-do feather in your hiking cap, but it is the most difficult hike in this entire guidebook. The rock scramble and the elevation gain have everything to do with this rating.

Despite the challenges, this hike is popular to the extreme. If you can, save your trek for a weekday. But hiking it on a weekend is better than not hiking it at all. Strike up the north slope of the mountain, then emerge onto a massive granite slab with incredible panoramas. Enter a maze of boulders, with some bona fide rock scrambling to reach the summit. The views are among the best in the park. Leave the rugged mountaintop, and reenter the lowlands along the pretty valley of Brokenback Run on a foot-relieving gravel fire road.

Best Time

This very busy hike is best done on clear, dry weekdays, not only to minimize crowding and maximize views, but also for safe hiking. The loop requires a challenging rock scramble that could become hazardous in wet or icy conditions. Also, be apprised pets are not allowed on half the hike, so please leave your dog at home on this trek.

TRAIL USE
Day Hiking,
Pets Prohibited

LENGTH
9.1 miles, 6–8 hours

VERTICAL FEET
±2,425'

DIFFICULTY
- 1 2 3 4 **5** +

TRAIL TYPE
Loop

START & FINISH
N38° 34.297'
W78° 17.346'

FEATURES
Summit
Ridgeline
Stream
Autumn Colors
Wildflowers
Great Views
Geological Interest

FACILITIES
Restrooms at trailhead

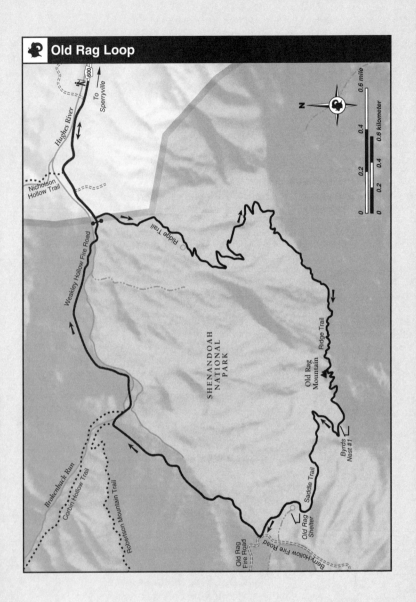

To Sperryville

Hughes River

Nicholson Hollow Trail

Weakley Hollow Fire Road

Ridge Trail

SHENANDOAH NATIONAL PARK

Old Rag Mountain

Ridge Trail

Byrds Nest #1

Saddle Trail

Brokenback Run

Corbin Hollow Trail

Robertson Mountain Trail

Old Rag Shelter

Old Rag Fire Road

Berry Hollow Fire Road

N

0.2   0.4   0.6 mile

0.2   0.4   0.6 kilometer

Finding the Trail

From the intersection of US 211 and US 522 in Sperryville, take US 522 south for 0.8 mile to VA 231. Turn right on VA 231 and follow it 8 miles to VA 601, Peola Mills Road. Turn right on VA 601, and follow it 0.3 mile, cross the Hughes River, then veer right, staying with VA 601. Stay with the blacktop as it becomes Nethers Road and leads up the Hughes River Valley to the lower Old Rag parking lot at 3.3 miles. Park here.

Alternative directions: From the intersection of US 29 Business and VA 231 in Madison, take VA 231 north for 12.4 miles to VA 602, Nethers Road. Follow VA 602, and stay with Nethers Road for a total of 3.4 miles from VA 231 to reach the lower parking lot.

Old Rag is Virginia's contribution to the great mountains in America.

Trail Description

The hike starts with a road walk. Leave the lower parking area ▶1 and walk up the pavement of quiet VA 600, passing the Nicholson Hollow Trail at 0.5 mile. Make the upper parking area at 0.8 mile. ▶2 Head left on the Ridge Trail, officially entering the national park. The climb innocently starts beneath cove hardwoods on a wide, uniform slope. Trailside boulders give a hint of things to come. The path switchbacks a couple of times, then ascends along a small, boulder-strewn hollow. Sharply turn away from the hollow at 1.8 miles, rising through chestnut oaks, sassafras, and gum. More switchbacks diminish the slope's steepness. Pass a tiny rill at 2.5 miles. Still more switchbacks twist ahead. The trail levels off at 2.8 miles. Weary hikers rest at this point. The Ridge Trail turns sharply right, climbing more. Ascend onto a granite slab. Your initial panoramas open. ▶3

The next mile is incredible, and incredibly challenging. Follow the blue blazes over, under, and around boulders, crevices, and outcrops. It

Autumn Colors

Ridgeline

Great Views

Geological Interest

takes both hands and feet across bare, steep rock to achieve the peak. Intermittent wooded stretches break up the climb. It's challenging and exciting—you will use all fours. At times, the scramble seems like a grand, granite maze. Be careful and keep following the blue blazes painted on rock. Take your time to visit outlying granite openings to absorb views of the nearby summit you are scaling, the surrounding mountains, and the lowlands beyond.

Level off at 3.6 miles, on the rocky shoulder of Old Rag. More stone stands between you and the summit, which you reach at 3.9 miles. ▶4 A few rocks to your right create the high point at 3,268 feet. Wind-sculpted vegetation clings to life among the cracks and crevices. Certain areas are cordoned off to protect this vegetation. Find your favorite overlook and take a well-deserved break.

 Summit

 Great Views

Start down the Saddle Trail, which veers away from the peak through heavily canopied woodland. Make your way off the west slope of Old Rag, passing outcrops with views directly to Robertson Mountain. Reach stone Byrds Nest Shelter #1, located in a saddle, at 4.4 miles. ▶5 It is for day-use only, but would be convenient in a storm.

Continue switchbacking down in sharply sloped woods. Come to Old Rag Shelter at 5.4 miles. ▶6

Old Rag Loop Elevation Profile

Opposite: *This hike takes you through some tight squeezes.*

The wooden shelter is day-use only too. A short path leads to a reliable spring. Leave the shelter on a wide fire road. The easy hiking is a relief and contrasts completely with your ascent. Drift into a trail junction and gap filled with tall pines and hardwoods at 5.8 miles. ▶7 Turn right here, and head down the Weakley Hollow Fire Road.

After a sharp right on the fire road, you pass the Robertson Mountain Trail at 6.9 miles. Brokenback Run noisily cuts through the valley you have entered. Just past this intersection the Corbin Hollow Trail heads left. Keep straight, spanning Brokenback Run on a metal bridge at 7.1 miles. ▶8 As you walk the road, look for the large, 18- to 24-inch leaves of the umbrella magnolia tree. The unmistakable leaves are pointed at both ends. This tree prefers low-elevation streamside environments. Look also for some huge rock piles from pioneer days.

Cross Brokenback Run again on three footbridges at 8.2 miles. Span a side stream on yet another footbridge, then complete the loop at the upper parking lot at 8.3 miles. ▶9 From here, backtrack to the lower lot, completing the hike at 9.1 miles. ▶10

Stream

Wildflowers 🌸

🚶 MILESTONES

▶1	0.0	Old Rag lower parking lot
▶2	0.8	Reach upper parking lot for Old Rag, and turn left on Ridge Trail
▶3	2.9	First vistas and rock scramble
▶4	3.9	Old Rag summit and join Saddle Trail
▶5	4.4	Byrds Nest Shelter #1
▶6	5.4	Old Rag Shelter
▶7	5.8	Right on Weakley Hollow Fire Road
▶8	7.1	Cross Brokenback Run on a metal bridge
▶9	8.3	Old Rag upper parking lot
▶10	9.1	Old Rag lower parking lot

Stony Man Loop

This hike traverses some of the highest terrain in the park. First you cruise a high-country nature trail and make a side loop to the summit of Stony Man Mountain, where cliffs rise 3,000 feet above the Shenandoah Valley and present superlative panoramas. You then take the Little Stony Man Trail to the peak of Little Stony Man, where more overlooks await. Your return trip is along the Passamaquoddy Trail, with still more views. Hike along the North Slope of Stony Man Mountain to reach Furnace Spring, which once was used in a copper-mining operation. Climb through mixed evergreens and hardwoods back to the trailhead, completing this highlight-laden loop.

TRAIL USE
Day Hiking,
Pets Prohibited
LENGTH
3.4 miles, 2–3 hours
VERTICAL FEET
±800'
DIFFICULTY
– 1 2 **3** 4 5 +
TRAIL TYPE
Loop
START & FINISH
N38° 35.581'
W78° 22.548'

FEATURES
Summit
Ridgeline
Autumn Colors
Wildflowers
Great Views
Historical Interest
Geological Interest

FACILITIES
Nearby Skyland Resort

Best Time

This high-country hike will be cool even in summer. Yet you can best enjoy the views whenever the skies are clear, primarily spring and fall. Be apprised that the loop is busy on fair-weather summer weekends.

Finding the Trail

This hike starts near the north entrance to Skyland Resort off Skyline Drive. At the turn you will see a sign indicating that this is the highest point on Skyline Drive; this turn is located at milepost 41.7. Immediately after turning toward the Skyland Resort, turn right into the parking area for the Stony Man Trail.

Stony Man Loop

Little Stony Man

To Thornton Gap

Skyline Drive

Passamaquoddy Trail

S. Fork Dry Run

Skyland Fire Road

Furnace Spring

Stony Man

Hemlock Springs Overlook

Furnace Spring Trail

Stony Man Horse Trail

Skyland Road

Skyland Area

Skyland Resort

41
7

SHENANDOAH NATIONAL PARK

Skyline Drive

Bridle Trail

Skyline Drive

To Swift Run Gap

Whiteoak Canyon Trail

N

0   0.1   0.2   0.3 mile

0   0.1   0.2   0.3 kilometer

Trail Description

The beginning of this hike can be a little confusing.
▶1 Here, a sign indicates the path as the Stony Man
Trail; this, however, is also the Appalachian Trail
(AT)—the two run in conjunction here. You can
purchase an interpretive booklet at the trailhead
to enhance your nature-trail experience. Walk a
pleasant pea-gravel path amid fern gardens overlaid
by hardwoods. Preserved hemlocks add a touch of
evergreen to the woods. Later you will also see a few
spruce trees.

Autumn Colors

Ridgeline

At 0.4 mile, come to an intersection. ▶2 This
is the highest point on the AT in Shenandoah
National Park—3,837 feet. But you are fixing to
get even higher. Turn left, still ascending to make
the subloop to the summit of Stony Man, staying
with the nature trail. Split right ahead, following the
sequence of the interpretive posts. Note the squat,
wind-sculpted haw trees as you climb.

At 0.7 mile, reach a four-way trail intersection. Turn right toward the summit of Stony Man.
Incredible panoramas open ahead. ▶3 To your left,
you can see the Skyland Resort. Ahead lay Shenandoah
Valley and the town of Luray, Massanutten Mountain
running parallel to the Blue Ridge, and beyond that,
North Mountain forming the Virginia–West Virginia
state line. To your right, northerly, look below at
the upthrust cliffs of Little Stony Man and at Skyline
Drive and the park's North District. The name Stony
Man derives from this peak, the park's second high-
est point, looking like the face of a bearded man.
The Stony Man's face can be clearly seen from the
north on milepost 38.9 of Skyline Drive at Stony Man
Mountain Overlook.

Summit

Great Views

Return to the AT, and then resume a northbound direction. The trail drops steadily through
northern hardwoods, including cool-climate spe-
cialist yellow birch, on the east slope of the Blue
Ridge. Reach the tan cliffs of Little Stony Man at

Summit 1.7 miles. ▶4 More grand views open before you. Look up to Stony Man for Shenandoah visitors milling about and looking ant-sized. The jagged cliffs have an especially rugged appearance as they emerge from the surrounding forest. The squared-off fields of Shenandoah Valley below contrast with

Great Views the craggy mountains to your right.

Return to woods beyond the cliff, switchbacking downhill to make another trail junction at 1.9 miles. ▶5 Leave the white-blazed AT, and turn left on the Passamaquoddy Trail, blazed in blue. Soon pass beneath the cliffs of Little Stony Man on a path constructed with considerable effort from native stones. Open onto a lower outcrop that avails yet another overlook from which the west side of the Blue Ridge and Lake Arrowhead opens below. The rising slope of Stony Man Mountain is especially impressive. Begin meandering the northwest side of the peak on a steep slope; the well-constructed trail

Geological Interest makes hiking a breeze. Walk beneath cliffs. Come to a rock overhang and dripping spring at 2.4 miles. At 2.5 miles, reach your low point of 3,200 feet, then

Wildflowers begin a gentle uptick. Fire cherry trees rise where hemlocks once stood. Pass beneath a transmission line at 2.8 miles.

Reach Furnace Spring at 2.9 miles. ▶6 You can hear the water flowing behind a locked door.

Stony Man Loop Elevation Profile

The views from Stony Man *can make you feel small in the scheme of things.*

The old copper mine was in this vicinity and used the spring, but the shaft has since been filled in and no trail leads to it. Come to an intersection with Skyland Fire Road and the Furnace Spring Trail. Make a hard left here, joining the yellow-blazed Furnace Spring Trail, passing directly above Furnace Spring on a doubletrack. The path then narrows and reenters deep woods. Snake your way uphill in rocky forest. The trailbed is fainter here. Look for yellow blazes on the trailside trees amid more preserved hemlocks. Meet the Stony Man Horse Trail, and turn left, tracing it a short distance to reach the Stony Man Trail Parking Area and the hike's conclusion. ▶7

 Historical Interest

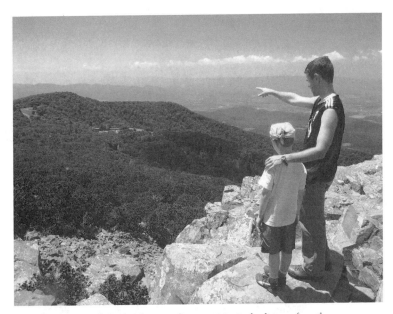

A father *points out Skyland and surrounding mountains in the distance from the crags of Stony Man.*

🚶 MILESTONES

▶1	0.0	Stony Man Trail Parking Area at milepost 41.7
▶2	0.4	Left toward Stony Man Summit
▶3	0.8	Stony Man Summit
▶4	1.7	Little Stony Man Summit
▶5	1.9	Passamaquoddy Trail
▶6	2.9	Left on Furnace Spring Trail
▶7	3.4	Stony Man Trail Parking Area at milepost 41.7

Robertson Mountain

Robertson Mountain is one of the park's best but least-visited scenic summits—most people pass it up to climb nearby Old Rag. But on the way to Robertson Mountain, you get to explore a highland cove and wetland on the all-access Limberlost Trail. You then join Old Rag Fire Road, where the walking is easy. A more traditional singletrack foot trail takes you the last mile to the outcrops of Robertson Mountain.

The crowds thin when you leave the Limberlost Trail, which offers an excellent short nature walk of 1.3 miles for anybody, including wheelchair-bound visitors. Be apprised, however, that the Limberlost Trail is closed to pets—alternatively, you could start farther north at the Whiteoak Canyon Trailhead (milepost 42.6), hike to Old Rag Fire Road, and then pick up the remainder of the hike as described here.

Best Time

The trek to the outcrops on Robertson Mountain can be enjoyed most when the skies are clear.

Finding the Trail

The Limberlost Trail Parking Area is at milepost 43 on Skyline Drive. The signed parking area is just a short distance down a road on the east side of Skyline Drive. It is 12.5 miles south of the Thornton Gap Entrance Station on Skyline Drive.

Trail Description

To begin, take the gravelly Limberlost Trail right from the parking area, ▶1 and enter a former

TRAIL USE
Day Hiking
LENGTH
6.8 miles, 3.5–5 hours
VERTICAL FEET
±1,080'
DIFFICULTY
– 1 2 3 **4 5** +
TRAIL TYPE
Out-and-back
START & FINISH
N38° 34.805'
W78° 22.879'

FEATURES
Summit
Ridgeline
Stream
Autumn Colors
Great Views

FACILITIES
None

hemlock forest that Skyland Resort founder George Freeman Pollock helped protect nearly a century ago. Unfortunately, the hemlock woolly adelgid did in most of the hemlocks, though a few are preserved. White oaks, yellow birch, mountain laurel, and even some apple trees round out the forest mosaic. Ferns carpet moister areas in the cool perched valley standing higher than 3,200 feet. The pea-gravel track gently meanders through this upper drainage of Whiteoak Run. Contemplation benches have been placed astride the path.

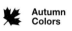 Autumn Colors

At 0.4 mile, traverse a boardwalk spanning an upland marsh. ▶2 Just ahead, the Crescent Rock Trail leaves right. Stay straight with the Limberlost Trail, passing through a former hemlock grove now being supplanted by bushy pin cherry trees. These transitional cherries will shade climax species, such as yellow birch, red spruce, and maybe hemlock when the forest reaches its full glory again, long after our lifetimes. At 0.8 mile, bridge a tributary of Whiteoak Run. At 0.9 mile, reach a four-way junction. ▶3 Here, the Whiteoak Canyon Trail leaves right for the cavalcade of cataracts that characterizes its lower reaches.

 Stream

Stay straight with the Limberlost Trail, shortly meeting Old Rag Fire Road. Turn right onto the yellow-blazed fire road where a sign reads HORSE PATH, SKYLAND, BIG MEADOWS. ▶4 The wide gravel track drops easterly, bridging Whiteoak Run at 1.1 miles. Stay left at a road split just ahead—this is where the horse concessionaire at Skyland turns around. The fire road climbs away from the stream to reach a trail junction at 1.4 miles. Stay left on Old Rag Fire Road. Just ahead, when a horse trail leads left, stay right. At 1.6 miles, you pass an old ranger station–turned–maintenance building on your right. ▶5

 Stream

 Ridgeline

Begin a protracted downgrade. Watch for sizable oak trees scattered amid the woods. The trail

One of many outcrops *providing views from Robertson Mountain*

turns sharply to the left and approaches the Corbin Mountain Trail at 2.2 miles. ▶6 Keep descending gently on Old Rag Fire Road past more big trees.

Pass Corbin Hollow Trail at 2.7 miles. ▶7 Begin looking for the blue-blazed Robertson Mountain Trail ahead, where you turn left at 2.8 miles. ▶8 Your descent is over. The serpentine footpath, contrasting with the gentle nature trail and the wide fire road, enters a laurel thicket and then turns back right. Look for the huge oak tree at the turn. You

Robertson Mountain Elevation Profile

curve around the green giant. It would take three hikers with arms outstretched to encircle it.

The real climbing doesn't start for another quarter mile, where the path switchbacks among rocks and trees, crowded by mountain laurel. It is hard to figure out which way the trail is going—except up. At 3.3 miles, the trail passes the summit on your right. Look on your right for a blue-blazed spur trail to the peak. The balance of the Robertson Mountain Trail leads straight. Take the spur past a grassy flat, ideal for picnicking, then continue on to the highest of several outcrops on Robertson Mountain. ▶9

 Summit

The depths of Whiteoak Canyon fall below. Look for the cleared overlooks along Skyline Drive and the Blue Ridge. The hump of Hawksbill Mountain looms tall to the southwest. Views to the north are a little harder to find, but scout around. Old Rag is to the east. Interestingly, Robertson Mountain, at 3,296 feet, is 5 feet higher than Old Rag. Take your time to let it all soak in; scout for more outcrops. It's great being on top of this mountain. On your return trip, near the trailhead, you can backtrack on the Limberlost Trail or take Old Rag Fire Road directly to the parking area.

 Great Views

	MILESTONES	
▶1	0.0	Limberlost Trail Parking Area
▶2	0.4	Crescent Rock Trail leaves right
▶3	0.9	Bisect Whiteoak Canyon Trail
▶4	1.0	Right on Old Rag Fire Road
▶5	1.6	Pass old ranger station on right
▶6	2.2	Corbin Mountain Trail leaves left
▶7	2.7	Corbin Hollow Trail leaves left
▶8	2.8	Left on Robertson Mountain Trail
▶9	3.4	Robertson Mountain summit

Falls of Whiteoak Canyon

Old Rag Fire Road

Whiteoak Fire Road

Upper Whiteoak Falls (No. 1)

Whiteoak Canyon

Tims River

Lower Whiteoak Falls

SHENANDOAH NATIONAL PARK

Whiteoak Canyon Trail

Whiteoak Run

Berry Hollow Fire Road

Cedar Run Link Trail

600

Cedar Run Trail

private property

Cedar Run

Cedar Run Trail

N

To Madison and 29

| 0 | | 0.2 | | 0.4 | | 0.6 mile |

| 0 | 0.2 | | 0.4 | | 0.6 kilometer |

Falls of Whiteoak Canyon

It's hard to keep track of all the falls at Whiteoak Canyon. There are six sequentially numbered falls. The count starts from the Blue Ridge and ends at the base of the canyon. To confuse matters further, this hike starts at the bottom of Whiteoak Run and heads upstream. Whether or not you correctly identify and number the falls, take this classic Shenandoah hike, for there are not only falls but also canyon views and everywhere-you-look beauty. However, beware the warm-weather weekend crowds. I highly recommend heading in a different direction during these times.

Best Time

Because this hike has no stream crossings, you can hike it in winter and spring without worry. That's when the falls are their boldest. In spring, wildflowers are their showiest. By all means, avoid this hike when it's crowded, on summer and fall weekends with nice weather.

Finding the Trail

From the town of Madison, on US 29 north of Charlottesville and south of Culpeper, drive north on VA 231 for 5 miles to VA 670. Turn left on VA 670, and follow it for 5 miles to VA 643. Turn right on VA 643, and follow it for less than a mile to VA 600. Turn left on VA 600, follow it 3.7 miles, and then turn left into the Berry Hollow Parking Area. The trailhead is in the back of the far parking area.

TRAIL USE
Day Hiking
LENGTH
5.2 miles, 3.5–4.5 hours
VERTICAL FEET
±1,400'
DIFFICULTY
– 1 2 3 **4** 5 +
TRAIL TYPE
Out-and-back
START & FINISH
N38° 32.370'
W78° 20.962'

FEATURES
Stream
Waterfalls
Wildflowers
Great Views
Steep
Geological Interest

FACILITIES
None

Trail Description

Waterfall lovers:

don't miss this hike.

Leave the rear of the parking area in Whiteoak Canyon, ▶1 and travel a trail easement through private property, reaching Cedar Run. At this point, the streambed is often dry, even though Cedar Run may be flowing upstream. Span Cedar Run on a metal bridge. Beech, sycamore, black birch, and magnolia shade the track. Ferns reflect the moist nature of a valley that is wide at this point and hasn't yet narrowed into a canyon.

When you reach the Cedar Run Trail junction at mile 0.2, ▶2 veer right, staying on the Whiteoak Canyon Trail. The Cedar Run Trail leads left for its own series of falls on an ultra-rocky path. Bridge Whiteoak Run, a rocky river if there ever was one. The sandy trail gently ascends along the right bank of the creek. Sycamores overhang the stream. The rock walls and piles are evidence that this area was once cultivated.

Stream

Come directly alongside the stream and reach the junction with the Cedar Run Link Trail at 0.8 mile. ▶3 Backcountry camping is prohibited beyond this point. Beyond here, the terrain is steep and rocky and not suitable for pitching a tent. Stay on the east bank of Whiteoak Run, entering a rock garden. The canyon closes. The stream begins gathering in deep pools. The path becomes correspondingly rockier

Falls of Whiteoak Canyon Elevation Profile

and steeper. Rock-hop the Tims River, which has a falls of its own, on your right. Just beyond this crossing, close in on Lower Whiteoak Falls (Number Six) at 1.4 miles. ▶4 A short trail leads left to the precipitous two-tier, 60-foot falls, which spills over an open rock face. The uppermost falls, where this hike ends, is the canyon's tallest at 86 feet. The ones in between—that are hard to count because their tops and bottoms are indiscernible—purportedly range between 45 and 65 feet each.

Waterfall

The main trail switchbacks, meandering far away from the stream. The area can be confusing because erosive user-created trails continue straight up the canyon. Follow the switchbacks on the proper trail. Climb sharply along the base of a bluff in pines, well above the stream, sometimes traversing open rock. In places, steps have been chiseled into this bare stone. At 1.7 miles, come to a cedar tree that guards a rock slab overlook into the canyon. Catch glimpses of the crashing falls below and the lands beyond the canyon. Continue switchbacking up the canyon and below other cliffs. The stream and path come together again by 1.9 miles. This is where the numbered falls get confusing. Just enjoy the cataracts and leave the counting to others.

Steep

Great Views

Begin a pattern of coming to a falls and then switchbacking away and uphill to the base of another falls. Huge walls rise beyond the stream. Pass an overhanging boulder on your right at 2.3 miles. Keep climbing through a wonderment of rock and water, where pools and cascades beckon you off the trail and to Whiteoak Run.

Waterfall

As you continue uphill, a melding of stone and concrete makes the pathway more hiker-friendly. A side trail leads left to the base of Whiteoak Falls (Number One) at 2.4 miles. ▶5 The main trail switchbacks to the right and passes a concrete trail marker indicating the halfway point of the Whiteoak Canyon Trail, with an attendant warning

Just one *of the many falls in Whiteoak Canyon*

Waterfall

for hikers that a shuttle is unavailable at the bottom of the canyon. Apparently, hikers have walked the Whiteoak Canyon Trail from Skyline Drive and decided they couldn't walk back up. Come to a rock observation point for Whiteoak Falls (Number One) at 2.6 miles. ▶6 You are on a large slab well above the second-highest falls in the park at 86 feet. It slides over bare rock in multiple stages bordered by hardwoods. Rest and enjoy these falls and the good view into the canyon below. On your return trip, try to count the falls. After all, Whiteoak Run has more falls per mile than any other stream in the park.

🚶 MILESTONES

►1	0.0	Whiteoak Canyon Trailhead
►2	0.2	Cedar Run Trail leaves left
►3	0.8	Cedar Run Link Trail leaves left
►4	1.4	Lower Whiteoak Falls (Number Six)
►5	2.4	Side trail to base of uppermost Whiteoak Falls (Number One)
►6	2.6	Whiteoak Falls (Number One) observation point

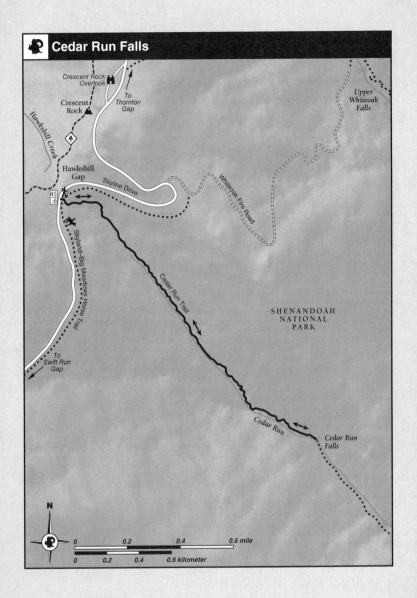

Cedar Run Falls

Crescent Rock Overlook

Crescent Rock

To Thornton Gap

Hawksbill Creek

Hawksbill Gap

Skyline Drive

45
.6

Whiteoak Fire Road

Upper Whiteoak Falls

Skyland–Big Meadows Horse Trail

Cedar Run Trail

SHENANDOAH NATIONAL PARK

To Swift Run Gap

Cedar Run

Cedar Run Falls

N

| 0 | 0.2 | 0.4 | 0.6 mile |

| 0 | 0.2 | 0.4 | 0.6 kilometer |

Cedar Run Falls

This hike leads you into rugged upper Cedar Run Canyon. The trail down to the falls is steep as it passes innumerable cascades spilling down the narrow boulder-laden gorge. This place is wild and deserving of national park protection. Your trip to the cascades will be slow because you need to watch your footing and stop often to admire the scenery.

Best Time

The falls are their boldest during winter and spring. Also, spring has flowers galore. More important, avoid this busy hike on nice weekends any time of year.

Finding the Trail

The Hawksbill Gap Trailhead is located at milepost 45.6 on Skyline Drive. The Cedar Run Trail starts behind the gravel parking area on the east side of Skyline Drive.

Trail Description

Leave the parking area and grassy Hawksbill Gap behind to enter tall hardwoods on the Cedar Run Trail. ▶1 Immediately come to a four-way trail junction. Keep forward, descending, still on the Cedar Run Trail. The Skyland-Big Meadows Horse Trail leaves left and right. Pass a rock outcrop often used as a relaxing locale for those returning up Cedar Run Canyon. The trail grade drops sharply in a thick forest alongside the upper reaches of Cedar Run.

TRAIL USE
Day Hiking

LENGTH
3.4 miles, 3–4 hours

VERTICAL FEET
±1,475'

DIFFICULTY
– 1 2 3 **4** 5 +

TRAIL TYPE
Out-and-back

START & FINISH
N38° 33.363'
W78° 23.197'

FEATURES
Stream
Waterfalls
Autumn Colors
Wildflowers
Steep
Geological Interest

FACILITIES
None

 Steep

155

Step over rock and wood waterbars that cut down on trail erosion. The white noise of cold mountain water serenades you all the way to the falls.

A northern hardwood forest of cherry, witch hazel, sugar maple, and large oaks rise from the stony woods. Despite elaborate trail work by the park service, the path remains very rocky. Take your time and carefully plant your feet—a rolled ankle is possible here. Sturdy boots and trekking poles will make the Cedar Run Trail more palatable. On the plus side: The plethora of boulders avails for ample resting spots on your return trip.

Cedar Run picks up steam on its drop, falling in multiple incarnations of moving water. A side branch crosses the trail, forming a cascade of its own. Soon, you walk alongside the fast-moving run. At 0.6 mile, step onto a wide rock, facing a cascade to your right. ▶2 Cedar Run descends 20 feet in a fan pattern and then crashes onto the rock on which you are standing.

Beyond this cascade the trail drops steeply alongside a stairstep cascade to your right and a rocky bluff to your left. At 0.9 mile, enjoy a brief interlude of level, relatively rock-free pathway. Then the trail resumes diving headlong into a cavalcade of stone and passes another slide cascade. At other times monstrous midstream boulders nearly obscure the water as it seeks gravity's level. At 1.1

Autumn Colors

Discover a wild, rocky canyon deserving of park protection.

Stream

Waterfall

Wildflowers

Cedar Run Falls Elevation Profile

Rock and water *combine to create scenes like this one in Cedar Run Canyon.*

miles, away from the stream, rock ramparts rise from the trees, forming canyon walls that echo and redouble the sounds of moving water. ▶3

At 1.3 miles, on the far side of the trail, a tributary stream adds its flow in a slide cascade. A deep pool with brook trout forms on Cedar Run just below this tributary. The clash of water and rock remains relentless. At 1.4 miles, pass another cliff line. ▶4 At 1.5 miles, the trail comes to a big, alluring pool below a two-tier cascade. ▶5 You have reached the crossing of Cedar Run. This is usually a rock-hop; however, it can be a wet crossing at high water.

You are now on the right-hand bank heading downstream. Yet the trail goes uphill, passing a feeder stream trickling in from your right. The Cedar Run Trail then descends a set of stone steps to the base of Cedar Run Falls at 1.7 miles. ▶6 The water

 Waterfall

 Waterfall

A clear pool *at the base of Cedar Run Falls*

spills down a slick rock face and lands in a deep and clear plunge pool, then it drops again in a whitewater froth through a narrow slot canyon. Many large boulders make good relaxing and observation points at this midfalls area. Half Mile Cliff rises on the far side of the falls.

Geological Interest

You can go a bit farther downstream to enjoy the lower segment of Cedar Run Falls. It has a deep plunge pool at the base of the slot canyon. You'll likely think of reasons to hang out down here since the hike back is ambitious (that is, very steep). Pace yourself, and use those trailside boulders to catch some air.

🚶	**MILESTONES**	
▶1	0.0	Hawksbill Gap Parking Area at milepost 45.6
▶2	0.6	Wide cascade
▶3	1.1	Trailside cliff line
▶4	1.4	Trailside cliff line
▶5	1.5	Cross Cedar Run
▶6	1.7	Cedar Run Falls

Hawksbill Summit

This moderately easy hike starts at a high elevation and gets to the top of things in Shenandoah. Along the way you enter a "sky island" of Canadian-type forest. Outcrops below the summit are just warm-ups for the nearly 360-degree view from the summit of Hawksbill. *Note:* Some of these outcrops are closed to the public, so please honor signed closures.

Best Time

Whenever the skies are clear is a good time to make Hawksbill. Since it is the park's highest point, Hawksbill receives heavy visitation, especially during summer.

Finding the Trail

The Upper Hawksbill Trailhead is on the west side of Skyline Drive at milepost 46.7. From the Thornton Gap Entrance Station, take Skyline Drive south for 15.2 miles to reach the parking area, on your right.

Trail Description

You get a jump on bagging this peak by starting out at higher than 3,600 feet, leaving less than 500 feet of vertical gain to the nose of Hawksbill. Leave from the back of the Upper Hawksbill Parking Area on the wide and gravelly Upper Hawksbill Trail. ▶1 Upland hardwoods of oak, birch, and maples line the track. Look for a few preserved hemlocks in the forest. Note how their lowermost branches grow in a ring of uniform height. This is a result of deer

TRAIL USE
Day Hiking
LENGTH
2.2 miles, 1.5–2 hours
VERTICAL FEET
±415'
DIFFICULTY
– 1 **2** 3 4 5 +
TRAIL TYPE
Out-and-back
START & FINISH
N38° 32.615'
W78° 23.591'

FEATURES
Summit
Autumn Colors
Great Views

FACILITIES
None

 Autumn Colors

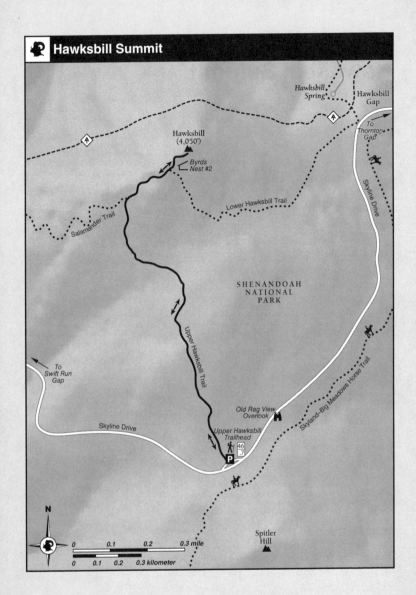

Hawksbill Spring

Hawksbill Gap

To Thornton Gap

Hawksbill
(4,050')

Byrds
Nest #2

Lower Hawksbill Trail

Salamander Trail

SHENANDOAH
NATIONAL
PARK

Skyline Drive

Upper Hawksbill Trail

To
Swift Run
Gap

Skyland-Big Meadows Horse Trail

Old Rag View
Overlook

Skyline Drive

Upper Hawksbill
Trailhead

46
7

P

Spitler
Hill

N

| 0 | 0.1 | 0.2 | 0.3 mile |

| 0 | 0.1 | 0.2 | 0.3 kilometer |

browsing—they can reach only so far up the tree, leaving this halo of greenery. The trail makes a quick jump and continues at a moderate grade. The small logs or waterbars across the trailbed help prevent erosion during prolonged rains and thunderstorms that sometimes wrack the Blue Ridge.

At this elevation the growing season is short; the trees don't begin to foliate until later May. Late September finds leaves turning a kaleidoscope of colors as trees prepare for a cold season that's significantly longer than that in the adjoining valleys. At 0.4 mile, the trail levels off then actually descends to join the old Hawksbill Fire Road at 0.6 mile.

Turn right and head up the former fire road, a wider track than the one you've been traveling. Begin to look for Fraser fir and red spruce, two northern climate species that are rare in Shenandoah and the Old Dominion. The evergreens are components of the Canadian-type (or boreal) forest that covered much of Shenandoah thousands of years ago. As the climate warmed and the ancient glaciers receded, these trees clung to the highest peaks of the Appalachians, where it was still cool enough for them to survive, forming "sky islands" of these Canadian plant communities.

At 0.9 mile, the Salamander Trail leaves left, and connects to the Appalachian Trail. ▶2 The main route to Hawksbill keeps straight and intersects the Lower Hawksbill Trail at 1.0 mile. ▶3 It leaves right for Hawksbill Gap. It seems that about everything in this vicinity is named Hawksbill.

Just ahead, come to a day-use shelter, Byrds Nest #2. It is a three-sided stone shelter, facing northwest. The refuge has a picnic table inside but the fireplace has been bricked shut. Camping is prohibited on the upper part of Hawksbill. Also, please respect signs indicating areas closed to the public on this special peak.

Hawksbill Summit Elevation Profile

Summit

Great Views

The main trail leaves right from the shelter. Ascend briefly, and then step up onto the summit of Hawksbill (4,050'). ►4 Though the exposed rocks provide good overlooks, the man-made observation platform bordered by a decorative stone wall may help you orient yourself. Metal plates showing the cardinal points are laid into the rock walls of the platform. You are standing atop the highest point in Shenandoah National Park. And what views you'll find: Old Rag in the eastern distance, Stony Man to the north, Skyline Drive and Crescent Rock nearby, and Nakedtop, as well as towns and hollows in the Shenandoah Valley to the west. While you're up here, please remember to honor outcrop closures in this fragile environment. It's a good feeling—being on top of the Blue Ridge.

🚶 MILESTONES

►1	0.0	Upper Hawksbill Trailhead at milepost 46.7
►2	0.9	Salamander Trail leaves left; stay right
►3	1.0	Hawksbill Trail leaves right to Hawksbill Gap Trailhead
►4	1.1	Hawksbill Summit at 4,050 feet

Rose River Falls Loop

This loop hike is long on beauty but sometimes short on solitude. Begin your trek on Rose River Fire Road, and gently descend to reach the lower Dark Hollow Falls Trail. Make the worthwhile 0.2-mile ascent to reach Dark Hollow Falls, while seeing other falls along this creek, Hogcamp Branch. Next, follow the Rose River Loop Trail downstream, passing numerous cascades along what is arguably the prettiest stream in the park. Bridge Hogcamp Branch, then pass the tailings of an old copper mine. Beyond here, the hike ascends the upper Rose River, passing Rose River Falls before returning to the trailhead.

TRAIL USE
Day Hiking,
Backpacking

LENGTH
4.0 miles, 2–3 hours

VERTICAL FEET
±830'

DIFFICULTY
– 1 2 **3** 4 5 +

TRAIL TYPE
Loop

START & FINISH
N38° 32.008'
W78° 25.257'

FEATURES
Stream
Waterfalls
Autumn Colors
Wildflowers
Historical Interest
Geological Interest

FACILITIES
None

Best Time

During spring the falls flow and the wildflowers grow. Summer and fall can be crowded. Hogcamp Branch, one stream along which you walk, can be a frozen delight in winter.

Finding the Trail

The Rose River Fire Road starts on the east side of Skyline Drive, just north of Fishers Gap Overlook at milepost 49.4. The parking is on the west side of the drive. The overlook is on a short, spur loop that leaves Skyline Drive. The Rose River Fire Road starts across Skyline Drive from the overlook's north end. From the Swift Run Gap Entrance Station, it is 16.1 miles to Fishers Gap Overlook.

Rose River Falls Loop

Blue Ridge

Hawksbill Creek

To Thornton Gap

Franklin Cliffs

Franklin Cliffs Overlook

Red Gate Fire Road

Skyland–Big Meadows Horse Trail

Fishers Gap

49
4

Fishers Gap Overlook

Rose River Falls

SHENANDOAH NATIONAL PARK

Skyland–Big Meadows Horse Trail

Rose River Fire Road

Skyline Drive

copper mine

Rose River

Rose River Loop Trail

Hogcamp Branch

Story Mountain Trail

Rose River Fire Road

Dark Hollow Falls Trail

To Swift Run Gap

Dark Hollow Falls

N

0   0.2   0.4   0.6 mile

0   0.2   0.4   0.6 kilometer

Trail Description

Pick up the gated Rose River Fire Road on the east side of Skyline Drive. ▶1 Walk a few feet down Rose River Fire Road, and reach an intersection. The Skyland–Big Meadows Horse Trail crosses the fire road. Keep straight on Rose River Fire Road, descending along the gravel track in a hardwood forest dominated by maple and white oak. Small rills flow off Big Meadows above, then pass under the fire road via culvert. The track levels out among locust trees, on land once farmed. Pass the Cave Cemetery on your right, atop a grassy hill at 0.5 mile. Watch for apple trees in this vicinity.

Historical Interest

Resume the descent. Hogcamp Branch falls loudly to your left. You soon walk along it. The forest canopy often opens along the roadbed, before reaching the junction with the Dark Hollow Falls Trail at a bridge over Hogcamp Branch at 1.0 mile. ▶2 Check out the 30-foot fall just above the bridge. A ribbon of frothing whitewater slices through a rock outcrop partially covered in moss. Turn right and head up the Dark Hollow Falls Trail. More falls tumble down as you head up, but you'll know Dark Hollow Falls. ▶3 It makes a wide drop, then gathers to tumble down three more tiers, a total descent of 70 feet. In summer the base of the falls can be crowded, since almost everyone has come from Skyline Drive on the Dark Hollow Falls Trail.

Waterfall

Return to Rose River Fire Road and cross the bridge. Just beyond the bridge, take the Rose River Loop Trail as it angles left and then downhill along Hogcamp Branch. ▶4 Young hardwoods are replacing woolly adelgid–killed hemlocks and—for now—Dark Hollow is dark no more. Hogcamp Branch puts on a scenic display while stairstepping down to meet the Rose River, falling and crashing in every type of fall, slide, cataract, and cascade, one tumbler after another, to gather in surprisingly deep pools, only to fall yet again. This is truly

 Stream

Dark Hollow Falls *spills over bedrock.*

national park–level scenery. Black and yellow birch and maple comprise the hemlock-less forest. At 2.0 miles, pass an open rock slab on the creek that lures hikers. A deep pool is at the base of the slab.

At 2.2 miles, reach a bridge spanning Hogcamp Branch. ▶5 The steel span arches well over and above Hogcamp Branch. The Rose River Loop then rock-hops a small stream. Reach the tailings of an old copper mine, with a path leading to the top of the tailings, back against a big bluff. Notice the stone and ironworks at the mine. This mine was

Historical Interest

Rose River Falls Loop Elevation Profile

opened in the early 1900s, but proved unprofitable and the shafts were filled. Keep downhill to reach a signpost near a large wooded flat. Turn left here and head upstream along the Rose River, which is crashing and dashing to your right, giving Hogcamp Branch a run for its scenic money.

 Stream

The Rose River Loop Trail leaves the river, climbing sharply in a fern forest, only to return at Rose River Falls at 2.8 miles. ▶6 Here, the water-course drops over a rock ledge about 25 feet, spreading out before reaching a pool. A spur trail leads downstream to a vista at lower Rose River Falls, which drops again as a narrow chute directly over a second ledge and out of sight from the view-ing spot, making a splash in a large pool.

 Waterfall

Beyond the falls, ascend a perched valley, under thriving hardwoods such as yellow birch and basswood. Reach another concrete signpost when meeting an old roadbed at 3.1 miles. Turn left here on a now-wide trail, leaving the river. Rise into drier, oak-dominated woods to meet the Skyland–Big Meadows Horse Trail at 3.6 miles. ▶7 Stay left here, as the two trails run in conjunction, mostly climbing to reach the Rose River Fire Road. It is but a few steps to Skyline Drive from here. Complete your loop at 4.0 miles. ▶8

🚶	**MILESTONES**	
▶1	0.0	North end of Fishers Gap Overlook at milepost 49.4
▶2	1.0	Right on Dark Hollow Falls Trail
▶3	1.2	Dark Hollow Falls
▶4	1.4	Cross Hogcamp Branch, and left on Rose River Loop Trail
▶5	2.2	Bridge Hogcamp Branch
▶6	2.8	Rose River Falls
▶7	3.6	Stay left at Skyland–Big Meadows Horse Trail
▶8	4.0	North end of Fishers Gap Overlook at milepost 49.4

Big Meadows Lodge

Blackrock

Lewis Spring Falls Trail

SHENANDOAH NATIONAL PARK

Hawksbill Creek

Lewis Spring Falls

Lewis Spring

Lewis Spring Service Road

Tanners Ridge Overlook

Big Meadows Campground

Big Meadows Area

Story of the Forest Trail

Big Meadows Road

Byrd Visitor Center

To Thornton Gap

Skyline Drive

Big Meadows Wayside

51 .4

Skyline Drive

Rapidan Road

N

To Swift Run Gap

| 0 | 0.1 | 0.2 | 0.3 mile |

| 0 | 0.1 | 0.2 | 0.3 kilometer |

Lewis Spring Falls Loop

Don't forget the camera or smartphone to capture the visual features along this hike that starts high and stays high. This loop takes place near the busy Big Meadows area, with its park lodge, visitor center, ranger station, and campground. Thus, this loop gets traffic, but deservedly so. Leave the parking area near Tanner Ridge Overlook, heading down Lewis Spring Service Road to reach the Appalachian Trail (AT). Walk northbound on the AT, climbing to Blackrock and its stellar views.

From there, the hike passes more interesting rock features, then joins the Lewis Falls Trail, where it descends to a loud, dramatic fall. Lewis Spring Falls is one of the highest elevation falls at Shenandoah. The distance is very doable, and the elevation changes aren't overly much, leaving you time to enjoy the other aspects of the greater Big Meadows area.

Best Time

In spring the falls rumble and the skies afford far-reaching views. Summer is good too, since this hike stays in the high country, but being near the main Big Meadows area can make it crowded. Fall can be busy too. Winter avails true solitude.

Finding the Trail

The parking area for the Lewis Spring Service Road is at milepost 51.4 on Skyline Drive. This parking area is sandwiched between the south entrance to Big Meadows and Tanners Ridge Overlook, on the

TRAIL USE
Day Hiking
LENGTH
3.3 miles, 2–3 hours
VERTICAL FEET
±850'
DIFFICULTY
– 1 2 **3** 4 5 +
TRAIL TYPE
Loop
START & FINISH
N38° 31.020'
W78° 26.502'

FEATURES
Summit
Ridgeline
Stream
Waterfall
Autumn Colors
Wildflowers
Great Views
Geological Interest

FACILITIES
Big Meadows Wayside
Campground
Lodge
Visitor center

west side of the road. The trailhead is 19.9 miles
south of Thornton Gap Entrance Station.

Trail Description

Leave the little parking area with several spots just
north of the Tanner Ridge Overlook. ▶1 Walk a few
yards north along Skyline Drive to reach the Lewis
Spring Service Road. Pass around a chain gate,
then head downhill on a gravel track bordered by
a stunted high-country forest of haw, fire cherry,
and maple, reclaiming former fields. Look for apple,

At high flows, *Lewis Spring Falls shoots a white froth over a rock face.*

birch, and locust trees too. The blue-blazed track crosses the yellow-blazed Tanners Ridge Horse Trail and continues descending.

At 0.2 mile, reach the AT. ▶2 Turn right here, heading northbound for Big Meadows Lodge. Lewis Spring is immediately below this intersection. Begin working uphill in hardwoods mixed with pines, even a preserved hemlock or two. Rocks and boulders of all sizes and descriptions are strewn about the forest floor. The well-used path features stonework to keep the trail from being sloped. At 0.7 mile, reach a spur trail leading right to Blackrock. ▶3 Turn right here and make the 0.1-mile climb to the outcrop, at 3,720 feet. ▶4

Along the way, see if you can find a few red spruce trees. In winter, they are easy to spot among the barren hardwoods. Mountain ash clings to the crags of Blackrock. The spiny rock protrusion opens to the west, where you can see the towns of Stanley and Luray in the Page Valley, amid the 180-degree view to the southwest and northwest, especially the high peaks of the park's North District. Below, the tops of oak trees seem close enough to touch. The AT can be seen below when the trees don't have leaves.

Return to the AT, curving below the rock massif of Blackrock. Another, smaller vista lies off the trail. Ahead, pass below the Big Meadows Lodge before meeting the Lewis Spring Falls Trail at 1.3 miles. ▶5 Here, turn acutely left on the Lewis Spring Falls Trail amid lush woods with a ferny understory. Continue downslope, looking for a level grassy spot near the trail good for picnicking, at 1.6 miles. Keep south along the western escarpment of the mountain, which drops off to your right. At 1.9 miles, the trail skirts below a lichen-covered rock protrusion.

Beyond here, the rocky trail steepens beneath the woods. Curve onto a southwest-facing slope, with mountain laurel and pines joining the sturdy oaks. Outcrops along the trail provide views into the

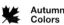
Autumn Colors

This hike starts high and stays high.

▲ **Ridgeline**

🔺 **Summit**

Great Views

Wildflowers

Geological Interest

Great Views

Stream

Waterfall

hollow of upper Hawksbill Creek, which becomes audible. Reach another junction at 2.5 miles. ►6 Here, a spur trail leads right to an outcrop and view into the valley below and lands beyond. Massanutten Mountain forms a backdrop. The main spur path crosses wide and rocky Hawksbill Creek and then curves beyond a precipice. A guardrail guides you the last bit to a rock-walled observation point. ►7 Here, you can look down at the 81-foot falls spilling over the rock face crashing into rocks and then splashing out of sight.

Backtrack to the Lewis Falls Trail, and begin a switchback-filled ascent along Hawksbill Creek, ►8 drifting into rich waterside woods and drier pine–oak forest away from the stream. Join an old roadbed, ►9 then pass Lewis Spring, which is housed in a rock-and-wood structure with a visible outflow. Just ahead, reach the AT again, at 3.1 miles. To your right is another boxed spring, and the site of the long dismantled Lewis Spring Shelter. From here, keep straight on the gravel road, backtracking to the trailhead. ►10

Lewis Spring Falls Loop Elevation Profile

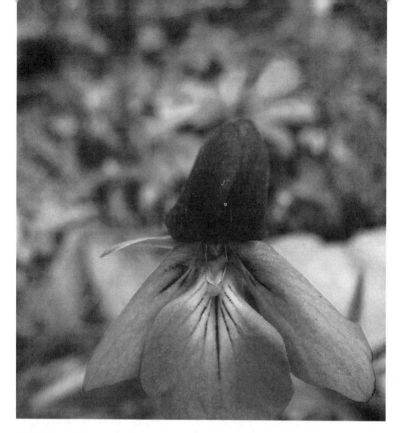

Delicate violet *graces the forest floor near Lewis Spring Falls.*

🚶 MILESTONES

▶1	0.0	Lewis Spring Service Road Parking Area at milepost 51.4
▶2	0.2	Right, northbound, on the AT
▶3	0.7	Spur to Blackrock
▶4	0.8	Vista from Blackrock
▶5	1.3	Acute left on Lewis Spring Falls Trail
▶6	2.5	Spur to vista and Lewis Spring Falls observation platform
▶7	2.6	Lewis Spring Falls observation platform and backtrack
▶8	2.7	Ascend along Hawksbill Creek
▶9	3.1	Complete loop at AT, and backtrack on Lewis Spring Service Road
▶10	3.3	Lewis Spring Service Road Parking Area at milepost 51.4

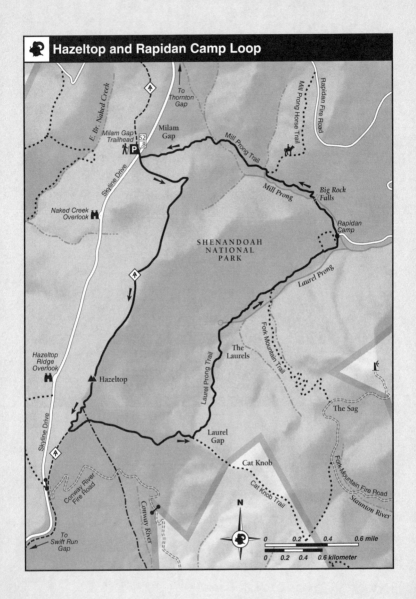

Hazeltop and Rapidan Camp Loop

To Thornton Gap

E. Br. Naked Creek

Milam Gap Trailhead

Milam Gap

Mill Prong Trail

Mill Prong Horse Trail

Rapidan Fire Road

Skyline Drive

Mill Prong

Big Rock Falls

Rapidan Camp

Naked Creek Overlook

SHENANDOAH NATIONAL PARK

Laurel Prong

Hazeltop Ridge Overlook

Hazeltop

Laurel Prong Trail

The Laurels

Fork Mountain Trail

The Sag

Skyline Drive

Laurel Gap

Fork Mountain Fire Road

Cat Knob

Conway River Fire Road

Cat Knob Trail

Staunton River

To Swift Run Gap

Conway River

N

0   0.2   0.4   0.6 mile

0   0.2   0.4   0.6 kilometer

Hazeltop and Rapidan Camp Loop

This loop takes you over Hazeltop, the third-highest peak in the park, and then traces attractive Laurel Prong Trail down to Rapidan Camp, the woodland getaway of President Herbert Hoover (1929–1933). There's much to see at the camp; you can even embark on a self-guided interpretive tour. Return to Milam Gap via Mill Prong Trail, and view Big Rock Falls along the way.

Best Time

This is a good summertime destination. The hike is shaded in greenery, and you can see historic Rapidan Camp at the time of year when President Herbert Hoover used it to escape the brutal summers in Washington, DC.

Finding the Trail

The Milam Gap Trailhead is located at milepost 52.8, on the west side of Skyline Drive. It can be reached by driving north on Skyline Drive for 12.7 miles from the Swift Run Gap Entrance Station. The Appalachian Trail (AT) is accessible behind the parking area. Start your hike here.

Trail Description

Head southbound on the AT from the Milam Gap Parking Area. ▶1 Note the preponderance of apple trees in this area. Bears gorge on them in fall. Cross Skyline Drive and come to a trail junction. To your left is Mill Prong Trail, your return route. Continue

TRAIL USE
Day Hiking,
Backpacking

LENGTH
7.2 miles, 6 hours
(includes 1 hour at
Rapidan Camp)

VERTICAL FEET
±1,300'

DIFFICULTY
– 1 2 3 **4** 5 +

TRAIL TYPE
Loop

START & FINISH
N38° 30.013'
W78° 26.759'

FEATURES
Summit
Ridgeline
Stream
Waterfall
Autumn Colors
Wildflowers
Wildlife
Great Views
Historical Interest

FACILITIES
None

 Wildlife

175

gently uphill, southbound on the AT through a forest shading fields of ferns, and reach a sharp right turn at mile 0.4. Now you are really going south as the AT heads toward Hazeltop.

The trail grade is nearly level, but it rises slightly on a slowly narrowing ridge. At points the AT is arrow-straight. Note the trailside upthrust rocks. At 1.9 miles, a spur leads right to a rocky overlook. ►2 Here, you can enjoy an open view to the west of the South Fork Shenandoah River Valley and waves of mountains in the distance. Achieve the peak of Hazeltop (3,812') at 2.0 miles. To your right is a gnarled oak next to a large embedded rock, the actual summit. To the left of the trail is a small balsam fir, a survivor of the forests that now thrive much farther north in New England and Canada. Its needles are flat, fragrant, and friendly (not sharp). Leave the summit, and come to a left turn. To your right are two red spruce trees, another member of the Canadian forest. Its needles are a darker green, rounded, and sharp. These trees grow in only a few locations in the park.

The AT drops moderately and approaches the scenic Laurel Prong Trail at mile 2.4. ►3 Turn left on Laurel Prong Trail. Several springs flow over the boulder-laden slope. The going is slow on the irregular tread. The Conway River Valley falls away to your right. The trail descends sharply, levels off,

Ridgeline ▲

Great Views 🔭

Summit 🔺

Visit one of America's first presidential retreats.

Hazeltop and Rapidan Camp Loop Elevation Profile

Rapidan Camp, *Herbert Hoover's presidential backcountry retreat*

and then makes a final dip to arrive at Laurel Gap and a trail junction at 3.4 miles. ►4 Cat Knob looms to the east. This is a good place to take a break—if the winds aren't howling.

Turn left, staying on the Laurel Prong Trail. It continues to drop sharply while snaking through "The Laurels," a concentration of mountain laurel and likely the inspiration for the stream's name. Backpackers find legal campsites along this section of trail, but remember, you can't camp within a half mile of Rapidan Camp. Pass a spring at 3.9 miles, the first of several rills flowing off Hazeltop. A few hemlock trees are hanging on. The valley forest is in transition. Rock-hop Laurel Prong at 4.1 miles. Watch for stone fences from pioneer farming days. At 4.7 miles, Fork Mountain Trail leaves right, ►5 into a thicket of rhododendron that is perhaps yet another inspiration for the stream's name;

Stream

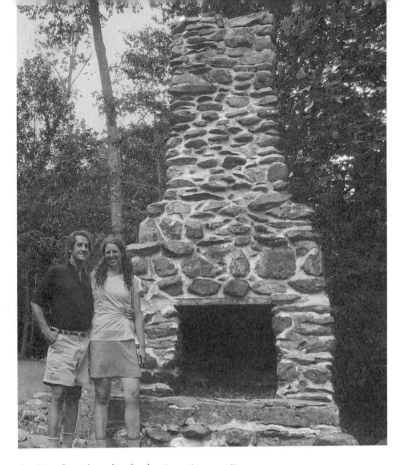

Rapidan Camp's *outdoor fireplace is a unique amenity.*

mountaineers often called rhododendron "laurel" and mountain laurel "ivy." Confusing, huh?

Continue straight on the Laurel Prong Trail. A spur trail leads left to Five Tents, the original dwelling site for Herbert Hoover. When the president first came here, workmen built five tents on platforms, around which a cabin was ultimately constructed. You can still see the fireplace. Arrive at Rapidan Camp at 5.3 miles. ▶6 Situated at the confluence of Laurel Prong and Mill Prong, the camp lies in a lovely wooded setting. Walk around, and check out the three buildings and interpretive information. There are short nature trails here too. This place

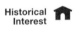

**Historical
Interest**

is engaging, so give it at least an hour. Imagine the president and his compadres strategizing on subjects of national import—trout fishing too. Back then hemlocks shaded and cooled the flat.

Continue your loop hike on the Mill Prong Trail, which starts near the Creel Cabin. Climb along the steep valley, rife with wildflowers in spring. The trail now drops to Mill Prong, crossing it below Big Rock Falls at mile 5.7. ▶7 Big Rock Falls slips 15 feet over a rock slide into a large, deep pool. President Hoover surely slung a fly rod here.

 Wildflowers

 Stream

 Waterfall

The trail switchbacks, levels off in a rocky section, and intersects the Mill Prong Horse Trail at mile 6.1. ▶8 Bear left, still on the Mill Prong Trail, crossing a side branch, and then rock-hop Mill Prong once more at 6.6 miles. ▶9 The stream is now wide, shallow, and pocked with stones. The path leads into an open, ferny forest. Enter a grassy glade before intersecting the AT at mile 7.2. ▶10 Turn right on the AT, cross Skyline Drive, and return to the Milam Gap Trailhead.

🚶 MILESTONES

▶1	0.0	Milam Gap Parking Area at milepost 52.8
▶2	1.9	Spur leaves right to overlook on Hazeltop
▶3	2.4	Left on Laurel Prong Trail
▶4	3.4	Left at Laurel Gap, still on Laurel Prong Trail
▶5	4.7	Fork Mountain Trail leaves right
▶6	5.3	Rapidan Camp
▶7	5.7	Big Rock Falls
▶8	6.1	Mill Prong Horse Trail leaves right
▶9	6.6	Cross Mill Prong
▶10	7.2	Meet AT and return to parking area

Staunton River Loop

Chapman Mountain

Rapidan Fire Road

Graves Mill Trail

Alt

662 P

Slide Cascade

Staunton River Trail

Doubletop Mountain

Rapidan Fire Road

Rapidan River

Rapidan Cabins

RAPIDAN WILDLIFE MANAGEMENT AREA

Staunton River

McDaniel Hollow Trail

Bear Church Rock

Rapidan Fire Road

Rapidan Camp

Fork Mountain

Jones Mountain Trail

Jones Mountain

RAPIDAN WILDLIFE MANAGEMENT AREA

Mill Prong Horse Trail

Big Rock Falls

Fork Mountain Trail

Laurel Prong Trail

Jones Mountain Trail

Mill Prong

Mill Prong Trail

Cat Knob Trail

Conway River Fire Road

Conway River

SHENANDOAH NATIONAL PARK

Milam Gap

To Thornton Gap

Skyline Drive

Laurel Prong Trail

Bootens Gap

55 P

To Swift Run Gap

0 0.3 0.6 0.9 kilometer
0 0.3 0.6 0.9 mile

N

Staunton River Loop

Best Time

This adventure follows—and crosses—two major park streams, making late spring–fall the best time to undertake the hike. Also, the waterways provide good swimming and fishing opportunities at that time. To make this a long day hike you will need the long daylight hours of summer.

Finding the Trail

The hike starts at the Bootens Gap Parking Area, milepost 55.1 on Skyline Drive. From the Swift Run Gap entrance station, take Skyline Drive north 10.6 miles to the trailhead, on the east side of Skyline Drive.

Trail Description

This can be a very long day hike but is better executed as a backpack. The circuit travels high and low, sporting mountaintop vistas as well as park history. However, most of the adventure is along the Staunton River and its mother stream, the Rapidan River. Both waterways deliver national park–level scenery. Staunton River has three noteworthy waterfalls with a host of other cataracts, while the Rapidan River is remarkable for its big pools framed by massive boulders and rock slabs. Expect a wide variance in trail conditions along the route. A portion of the hike traverses Rapidan Wildlife Management Area (WMA), where the hike traces a road open to vehicles. Other segments of the hike follow singletrack trails, old woods roads, and national park fire roads

TRAIL USE
Day Hiking,
Backpacking

LENGTH
18.6 miles, 9–11 hours

VERTICAL FEET
±2,825

DIFFICULTY
– 1 2 3 4 **5** +

TRAIL TYPE
Loop

START & FINISH
N38° 28.077'
W78° 27.443'

FEATURES
Ridgeline
Stream
Waterfall
Autumn Colors
Great Views
Swimming
Secluded
Historical Interest
Geological Interest

FACILITIES
Rapidan Cabins

open only to park personnel, as well as the venerable Appalachian Trail (AT).

The adventure leaves Bootens Gap, northbound on the AT. ▶1 A slight uptick leads you to the intersection with the stony Laurel Prong Trail at 0.4 mile. Turn right on the Laurel Prong Trail, ▶2 passing outcrops and emerging springs. Curve into Laurel Gap and a trail junction at 1.4 miles. Keep straight, joining the short but steep Cat Knob Trail, ▶3 huffing and puffing up a lesser-used path. Top out on a rock-slab trailbed, then mercifully descend to intersect the Jones Mountain Trail at 2.0 miles.

Turn left onto a seldom-trod segment of the Jones Mountain Trail, ▶4 wandering through a beautiful forest of maple, oak, and mountain laurel complemented with spreading ferns. All too soon, come to an interestingly named gap known as The Sag and a trail intersection at 2.9 miles. ▶5 Turn right on doubletrack Fork Mountain Fire Road, descending an easy route to meet the Staunton River Trail at 3.7 miles.

Conditions quickly change as you join the narrow, lesser-used, very rocky Staunton River Trail. ▶6 However, the water song of the plummeting Staunton River provides soothing background music under a mantle of yellow birch.

Difficult-to-reach cascades and cataracts testify to the steep gradient of the waterway as the trail teases hikers, coming near the waterway and turning away, at times traversing the side slope well above the dashing stream. At 4.7 miles, rock-hop crystalline Staunton River. Enter a flat with piled chestnut boards. ▶7 The place is called Hundley's Ford. Long ago the park service had these boards cut from trees killed by the chestnut blight. The hardiness of the boards testifies to the value of chestnut wood. Quickly cross the Staunton River a second time, joining an old woods road formerly used for training troops before World War II.

See the site of the first presidential retreat, used by Herbert Hoover.

Secluded

Autumn Colors

Secluded

Stream

This cataract *is called Gauge Rock Cascades by some.*

Here, where the valley flattens, was thickly inhabited during pre-park days—rock walls and piles were once borders for field and pasturage. Pass the McDaniel Hollow Trail near a massive boulder at 5.1 miles, then meet the other end of the Jones Mountain Trail at 5.5 miles. ▶8 At 6.2 miles a user-created spur trail heads left to a 12-foot slide cascade. At 7.1 miles, another spur trail leads left to a 20-foot cataract sometimes known as Jitterbug Falls. The white froth twists and turns atop a bare rock face into a plunge pool before pushing onward into shallows. Below Jitterbug Falls, the Staunton River frequently divides around islands, while the trail continues bisecting formerly settled lands. At 7.6 miles, pass above another waterfall just upstream of a USGS water gauge. You can see it from the trail above or walk down to its base and pool. This one—Gauge Rock Cascades—drops about 20 feet over a widening stone face.

Historical Interest

Waterfall

At 7.7 miles, the loop turns left on the Graves Mill Trail, ▶9 beginning its sojourn up the impressive Rapidan River. First you must rock-hop the Staunton River at its confluence with the Rapidan. Make an easy uptick on a wide track, Rapidan River gurgling to your right. Rock-hop the Rapidan at 8.8 miles. The river gradient and trail gradient both increase, and the famed boulders and pools of the Rapidan become prominent and commonplace. You will see them ahead for miles, beckoning you to pull up a rock and peer into their depths—or jump in, depending on the season. At 9.4 miles, join the Rapidan Fire Road. ▶10 Despite being inside Shenandoah National Park, this road is open to private vehicles, allowing access to Rapidan WMA, owned and managed by the State of Virginia.

Continue upriver, gently rising on the access road. At 11.0 miles, cross the road bridge over the Rapidan River. Enter Rapidan WMA. ▶11 Fork Mountain Fire Road enters to your left, near the primary Rapidan WMA parking area. Pass roadside campsites as you walk the gravel road. At 12.3 miles, come near the historic Rapidan Cabins, ▶12 an outlier of Rapidan Camp, also known as Camp Hoover. These cabins were used by staff during President Herbert Hoover's stays at the official camp upriver. You can rent these wood structures overnight. For more information, visit rapidancamps.org.

Stream

Swimming

Historical Interest

Staunton River Loop Elevation Profile

At 12.9 miles, reenter Shenandoah National Park, passing around a gate and leaving public auto access behind. The walking remains easy on the doubletrack. At 13.3 miles, Rapidan Fire Road leaves right. Head left toward Rapidan Camp, reaching a signed intersection at 13.8 miles. ▶**13** Split left on a foot trail to span Mill Prong via footbridge to reach Rapidan Camp, President Hoover's retreat to escape the torrid summers and even more torrid political climate in Washington, DC. Take time to view the buildings and read extensive interpretive information concerning this first presidential retreat, occupied during President Hoover's term, 1929–1933. During the warm season, on-site interpreters lead tours and answer questions. From the upper part of Rapidan Camp, pick up the slender Mill Prong Horse Trail. Climb along Mill Prong, shaded by deep forest. At 14.3 miles, rock-hop Mill Prong at Big Rock Falls, ▶**14** an 18-foot spiller sliding over a stone face. Keep climbing toward the Blue Ridge, reaching a junction at 14.8 miles. Angle left with the Mill Prong Trail. ▶**15** Up trail, cross a shallow section of Mill Prong, then rise through brushy forest. At 15.8 miles, meet the AT, near Skyline Drive at Milam Gap. Head left, ▶**16** southbound, on the AT, straddling the Blue Ridge. The hiking is easy as you stroll a long, straight, level parcel of Shenandoah National Park.

At 17.7 miles, a side path leads right to a stone outcrop providing a vista into the Shenandoah Valley and onward to West Virginia. ▶**17** Top out on Hazeltop at 3,800 feet before gently dropping to once again meet the Laurel Prong Trail at 18.2 miles. ▶**18** From here, backtrack 0.4 mile to Bootens Gap and the end of the hike. ▶**19**

 Historical Interest

 Stream

 Waterfall

 Geological Interest

 Ridgeline

Great Views

►1	0.0	Bootens Gap Parking Area, milepost 55.1, Skyline Drive
►2	0.4	Right on Laurel Prong Trail
►3	1.4	Laurel Gap, join Cat Knob Trail
►4	2.0	Left on Jones Mountain Trail
►5	2.9	Reach The Sag, right on Fork Mountain Fire Road
►6	3.7	Veer right on singletrack Staunton River Trail
►7	4.7	Reach two river crossings and piled chestnut boards at Hundley's Ford
►8	5.5	Pass other end of Jones Mountain Trail, falls ahead
►9	7.7	Left on Graves Mill Trail
►10	9.4	Left on Rapidan Fire Road
►11	11.0	Enter Rapidan WMA
►12	12.3	Pass Rapidan Cabins
►13	13.8	At historic Rapidan Camp, join Mill Prong Horse Trail
►14	14.3	Big Rock Falls
►15	14.8	Left on Mill Prong Trail, campsites in vicinity
►16	15.8	Left on Appalachian Trail, southbound
►17	17.7	Overlook
►18	18.2	Pass Laurel Prong Trail
►19	18.6	Bootens Gap Parking Area, milepost 55.1, Skyline Drive

Bear Church Rock via Staunton River

Bear Church Rock is one of the all-time top names in Appalachia. The origin is lost to time, but from the granite outcrop it doesn't take much imagination to visualize a pulpit overlooking the Staunton River Valley. The pulpit lies below the main granite crag where your views open. Conjuring up a bear preaching a sermon may prove more difficult, but some claim the panorama to be a near-religious experience. Your hike to the crag is rewarding too. The Staunton River tumbles in pools and cascades impressive for the limited stream volume. Be apprised that the nearly 2,000-foot elevation change is challenging.

Best Time

This hike is great year-round. The low-elevation trailhead makes it accessible in winter. You can enjoy streamside scenery without having to ford any streams. The Staunton River Valley presents wildflowers and cascades in spring and summer, while extensive views can be had from Bear Church Rock in autumn.

Finding the Trail

From US 33 Business in Stanardsville, east of Swift Run Gap, take VA 230, Madison Road, north for 7.1 miles to VA 662. Turn left on VA 662, Graves Mill Road. Follow VA 662 for 5.1 miles, then turn right onto Graves Road, which is still VA 662 (the road going forward here becomes VA 615). Immediately

TRAIL USE
Day Hiking,
Backpacking
LENGTH
7.6 miles, 4.5–5.5 hours
VERTICAL FEET
±1,950'
DIFFICULTY
– 1 2 3 4 **5** +
TRAIL TYPE
Out-and-back
START & FINISH
N38° 26.219'
W78° 22.003'

FEATURES
Ridgeline
Stream
Waterfall
Autumn Colors
Wildflowers
Great Views
Swimming
Secluded
Historical Interest
Geological Interest

FACILITIES
None

Bear Church Rock via Staunton River

Rapidan River

Graves Mill Trail

Graves Mill Trail

Graves Mill Trailhead

615

To Stanardsville and

33

SHENANDOAH NATIONAL PARK

Staunton River

Staunton River Trail

Wilson Run

Jones Mountain Cabin

Jones Mountain Trail

Staunton River Trail

McDaniel Hollow Trail

Bear Church Rock

Jones Mountain Trail

Staunton River

Garth Spring Run

McDaniel Hollow

RAPIDAN WILDLIFE MANAGEMENT AREA

649

N

0.6 mile
0.4
0.2
0

0.6 kilometer
0.4
0.2
0

bridge Kinsey Run, and follow Graves Road to dead-end at the Graves Mill Trailhead at 1.2 miles.

Trail Description

Leave the VA 615 trailhead on the Graves Mill Trail, passing around vehicle barrier boulders. ▶1 The Rapidan River rushes to your right. This is a popular fishing area, and you may see anglers along the many pools on the river. Make an easy trek up a nearly level valley, under towering hardwoods dominated by black birch, sycamore, and beech, with an odd cedar thrown in. Ferns are scattered across the forest floor.

At 0.5 mile, go left on the Staunton River Trail. ▶2 The Staunton River, a major mountain tributary of the Rapidan River, forms east of the Blue Ridge below Fork Mountain. By this point it is a full-fledged mountain cataract with alternating rapids and pools. The trail gradient increases, and you soon come alongside the Staunton River just in time to view a 15-foot slide cascade spilling over a rock slab. You can reach it on a short spur trail.

The Staunton River Trail continues up the wide, sloped valley, once cultivated by mountaineers, but now growing spring wildflowers under cucumber magnolias and tulip trees. Rock piles are especially visible when the leaves are off. Step over possibly

Bear Church Rock is a difficult and remote destination.

 Stream

 Autumn Colors

 Swimming

 Waterfall

Wildflowers

Bear Church Rock via Staunton River Elevation Profile

Even snakes *enjoy the waterfalls at Shenandoah National Park.*

dry Wilson Run at 0.9 mile. Continue up the valley in tight but spindly tree stands broken up by larger, more robust woods. At 1.3 miles, bisect a pair of huge boulder gates. ▶3 Leap rocky overflow braids from the Staunton River as well as rivulets flowing off Jones Mountain above you. Yellow birches appear as the path gains elevation. At 1.8 miles, watch for the foundations of an old-home site on your left, with many rock piles and stone fences as well.

Historical Interest

At 2.6 miles, the hike veers left onto the Jones Mountain Trail. ▶4 The ascent escalates, and watery sounds fade along the boulder-strewn hillside. Intersect the McDaniel Hollow Trail at 3.0 miles, following a short but steep burst. ▶5 Stay left with the Jones Mountain Trail, curving through tunnels of mountain laurel. The path levels off and then

Steep

meets the Jones Mountain Cabin spur trail at 3.3 miles. ►6 The dwelling, once home to pre-park resident Harvey Nichols, is available for overnight rental. It is maintained by the Potomac Appalachian Trail Club. For rental information visit patc.net.

Resume climbing toward Bear Church Rock, switchbacking up the east end of Jones Mountain. Reach a trail split at the crest of Jones Mountain. Turn right here and emerge onto multiple granite outcrops, broken by windswept trees clinging to crevices. ►7 The escarpment exposes the park's glory. Fork Mountain, Doubletop Mountain, and the crest of the Blue Ridge stand out. The rocky cone of Old Rag peeks above nearby ridges. Below, Staunton River and its tributaries carve a wooded valley. Both bears and hikers are rewarded on Bear Church Rock.

 Ridgeline

 Geological Interest

 Great Views

⚐	MILESTONES	
►1	0.0	Graves Mill Trailhead
►2	0.5	Left on Staunton River Trail
►3	1.3	Boulder gates
►4	2.6	Left on Jones Mountain Trail
►5	3.0	McDaniel Hollow Trail leaves right
►6	3.3	Spur to Jones Mountain Cabin
►7	3.8	Bear Church Rock

Bear Church Rock from Bootens Gap

Bear Church Rock from Bootens Gap

This solitude-laden high-country hike leads along the ridge of Jones Mountain to an incredible view from Bear Church Rock. The hiking along Jones Mountain is some of Shenandoah's finest. You are above 3,000 feet most of the hike, yet the trail is never steep for long and is level much of the way, making it about the easiest 9 mountain miles you can ask for. The whole hike is on hiker-only foot trails, meandering through varied and beautiful forests. It is a great way to spend a day in Shenandoah. Make sure to bring water.

Best Time

This hike is great during all seasons. You can experience clear views in fall, winter, and spring, while summer avails cool temperatures. Solitude can be found anytime.

Finding the Trail

Bootens Gap is located at milepost 55.1 on Skyline Drive. From the Swift Run Gap Entrance Station, head north on Skyline Drive for 10.4 miles to the Bootens Gap Parking Area. The small parking area will be on your right, the east side of Skyline Drive. Pick up the Appalachian Trail (AT) here.

Trail Description

Walk just a few steps down Conway River Fire Road, ▶1 then reach the AT. Turn left, northbound, as the AT ascends moderately up the southwest

TRAIL USE
Day Hiking
LENGTH
9.4 miles, 5–6.5 hours
VERTICAL FEET
±800'
DIFFICULTY
– 1 2 3 **4** 5 +
TRAIL TYPE
Out-and-back
START & FINISH
N38° 28.106'
W78° 27.446'

FEATURES
Ridgeline
Autumn Colors
Great Views
Secluded
Geological Interest

FACILITIES
None

Stay above 3,000 feet nearly the entire hike.

Geological Interest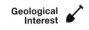

Ridgeline ▲

Autumn Colors 🍁

side of Hazeltop, coming to a trail junction at 0.4 mile. ►2 Turn right on the Laurel Prong Trail. The footbed descends past several springs on a boulder-laden slope, flowing from Hazeltop. The trail drops sharply just before arriving at breezy Laurel Gap and another trail junction at 1.4 miles. ►3 Keep straight, joining the short Cat Knob Trail. Follow the faint footbed uphill, twisting and turning among impressive gray boulders. Enter a slice of the Rapidan Wildlife Management Area at mile 1.8.

The trail makes one last jump and then descends slightly before intersecting the Jones Mountain Trail at 2.1 miles. ►4 It has come up 0.8 mile from The Sag, a simple but memorable Appalachian landmark name. Veer right, now on the Jones Mountain Trail.

The ridge-running path makes for pleasant walking among windswept oaks. The fern and grass understory, mingled with mountain laurel, adds more appeal. A sense of seclusion overwhelms the ridgeline. The little-used trail descends, making an unexpected right at mile 2.4. Come to a gap in a broken forest. Brush may crowd the path in late summer. Reenter the park at mile 2.7 in oak woodland. Begin an extensive, level stretch, trending slightly downhill. The scenery is among Shenandoah's finest.

In a grassy gap at mile 3.6, the trail turns left and down, east toward Bear Church Rock and away

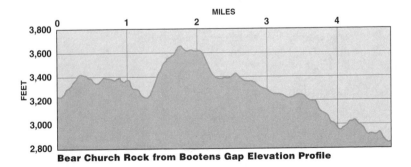

Bear Church Rock from Bootens Gap Elevation Profile

from Bluff Mountain. ▶5 Look for an outcrop on your left with warm-up views of Fork Mountain. Begin a more-down-than-not roller-coaster ride along Jones Mountain. Large granite outcrops rise among the hardwoods.

At mile 4.6, the trail zigzags very steeply down the point of the ridge among brush and laurel. Watch for a side trail splitting left in 0.1 mile. This side trail emerges onto the granite slab of Bear Church Rock. ▶6 The sloping rock creates a natural viewing platform. Look for water-filled potholes in the near and mountains aplenty in the far. What a perch!

 Great Views

From here, you can see Fork Mountain, Doubletop Mountain, and the crest of the Blue Ridge. The Staunton River Valley cuts a chasm below. This is one of my favorite overlooks in the entire park, and I have never seen a soul while up here. Explore the various outcrops broken by screens of vegetation, as well as the base of the outcrops. Make sure to allow plenty of time to return.

 Secluded

🚶	MILESTONES	
▶1	0.0	Bootens Gap Parking Area at milepost 55.1
▶2	0.4	Right on Laurel Prong Trail
▶3	1.4	Join Cat Knob Trail
▶4	2.1	Pick up Jones Mountain Trail
▶5	3.6	Turn left, away from Bluff Mountain
▶6	4.7	Bear Church Rock

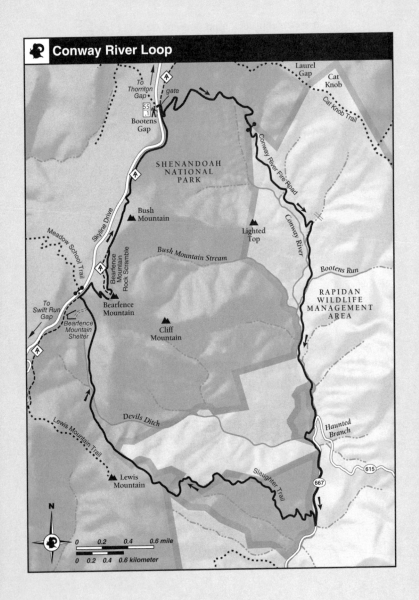

To
Thornton
Gap

gate

55
1

Bootens
Gap

Laurel
Gap

Cat
Knob

Cat Knob Trail

SHENANDOAH
NATIONAL
PARK

Conway River Fire Road

Bush
Mountain

Skyline Drive

Meadow School Trail

Bearfence
Mountain
Rock Scramble

Bearfence
Mountain

To
Swift Run
Gap

Bearfence
Mountain
Shelter

Lighted
Top

Conway River

Bush Mountain Stream

Bootens Run

RAPIDAN
WILDLIFE
MANAGEMENT
AREA

Cliff
Mountain

Devils Ditch

Lewis Mountain Trail

Lewis
Mountain

Haunted
Branch

615

Slaughter Trail

667

N

0   0.2   0.4   0.6 mile

0   0.2   0.4   0.6 kilometer

Conway River Loop

This loop leaves the Blue Ridge and follows the scenic Conway River through a parcel of the Rapidan Wildlife Management Area. Leave the Conway River, and head into the high country on the seldom-trod Slaughter Trail, passing a pioneer homesite, for the upper reaches of Devils Ditch. Complete your trip by clambering over Bearfence Mountain, with its 360-degree views, on a short but challenging rock and boulder scramble; pets are prohibited on this scramble. This loop makes for a long day hike but a great one- or even two-night backpack.

Please note that Rapidan Wildlife Management Area (WMA), managed by the State of Virginia, has hunting as well as different camping rules from Shenandoah National Park, so consult the latest information at the Virginia Department of Game and Inland Fisheries website (dgif.virginia.gov). Note also that both the Conway River Fire Road and the Slaughter Trail receive limited maintenance and may be overgrown in summer.

Best Time

This challenging loop has it all: views, waterfalls, streams, and ridges—something for every season. Spring affords extensive vistas, wildflowers, and bold streams, but it is double-edged since the hike requires three fords of the Conway River. Summer is cool on the river, and fall presents colors and even lower water. The views from atop Bearfence Mountain are boundless after the first cold fronts move through. Winter can be tough when it comes to the stream crossings.

TRAIL USE
Day Hiking,
Backpacking,
Pets Prohibited

LENGTH
12.0 miles, 7–9 hours

VERTICAL FEET
±2,300'

DIFFICULTY
− 1 2 3 4 **5** +

TRAIL TYPE
Loop

START & FINISH
N38° 28.106'
W78° 27.446'

FEATURES
Ridgeline
Stream
Waterfall
Autumn Colors
Wildflowers
Old-Growth Forest
Great Views
Historical Interest
Geological Interest

FACILITIES
None

197

Finding the Trail

The Conway River Fire Road starts at Bootens Gap at milepost 55.1 on Skyline Drive. From the Swift Run Gap Entrance Station, head north on Skyline Drive for 10.4 miles to the Bootens Gap Parking Area. The small parking area will be on your right on the east side of Skyline Drive. Conway River Fire Road starts in the back of the parking area.

Trail Description

Leave the Bootens Gap Parking Area on Conway River Fire Road. ▶1 The wide, grassy track makes two switchbacks before coming to the upper Conway River. It may be dry here in fall. Dive deeper into the valley, where bigger hardwood trees rise.

Autumn Colors

Pass through a gate at 1.4 miles, and enter the Rapidan WMA. ▶2 Red blazes mark the boundary between the national park and the wildlife area. Swing back left and cross an often-dry ravine at mile 1.6. Over the next couple of miles you may see a 4WD vehicle on the track. Rough 4WD roads splinter off the main path. Step over a fair-sized stream at mile 2.2, then come to another decent-sized but unnamed stream at 2.6 miles. ▶3 A 25-foot wet-weather fall tumbles in stages about 40 yards upstream from the trail (roadbed) you are on. Follow this tributary downstream.

Waterfall

Arrive at a fork in the road at 2.8 miles. The left fork leads to a large clearing. Stay on the right fork, leading to Bootens Run at 3.3 miles. Rock-hop Bootens Run, then come alongside the boulder-strewn Conway River. The trout-filled, boulder-laden, large watercourse presents everywhere-you-look beauty. The national park is on the far side of the stream.

Stream

At 3.8 miles, come to a concrete Shenandoah National Park trail signpost. ▶4 Here, VA 615 leads left. Stay right on the Conway River Fire Road, and shortly come to your first crossing of the Conway River. It should be a simple rock-hop in summer and fall, but can be a ford in winter and spring. Make your way carefully across the river, leaving any potential jeep traffic behind.

The Conway River, with its deep pools for fishing or wading, is now on your left. Travel a riverside rocky track under dense forest. At 4.4 miles, reach a wide flat with rock piles, indicating former farmland. Rock-hop Devils Ditch at mile 4.8. ▶5 As with most Shenandoah streams, flow can range from a trickle to a torrent. Pass a Rapidan WMA hunting trail that leads right, up the Devils Ditch.

Wildflowers

Come to another ford of the Conway River at mile 5.0. ▶6 Big boulders and deep water make this ford tough during high water, so exercise caution when crossing the stream here—hiking sticks help greatly. The trail leads uphill under scads of white pines, then descends back to the Conway. Come to your third and final river crossing at 5.5 miles. ▶7 This deep pool is a great summertime swimming hole. Cross the river here; this ford will likely get you wet, yet it's easier than the one just upstream. VA 667 is just 0.3 mile down a jeep road after the river crossing.

Stream

Come to the concrete signpost for the Slaughter Trail, and begin heading upstream. You will be in Shenandoah National Park the remainder of the hike. The Conway River should now be on your right. The rocky Slaughter Trail briefly parallels the Conway. Look for the rock walls and exotic bushes of an old riverside homesite. The Slaughter Trail leaves the river, climbing steeply up a spur ridge leading toward Lewis Mountain. Notice the old-growth white pines above you.

Historical Interest

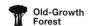
Old-Growth Forest

The path switchbacks left at mile 5.7 and then steepens even more before leveling off at mile 6.5. Congratulations—you have just climbed 850 feet in 1 mile. Traverse a gap, pass a rock pile, climb a little more, and then come to a homesite on your right. The chimney and foundation are crumbling. A spring is on the far side of the homesite. You might want to rest and explore the homesite because more climbing lies ahead.

Historical Interest 🏠

Keep ascending on the eroded trail, passing blazed boundary trees. Pass the ruins of an outbuilding on your left and a split-rail fence on your right. At mile 7.3 beneath a yellow birch, a rock-lined spring sends forth cool water. The moss- and grass-covered trail nears Lewis Mountain and levels out at mile 7.7. Watch as an old road leaves left for the crest of Lewis Mountain. Cruise along the east slope of the mountain, earning a little rest after

Stream 🏞️

climbing 1,750 feet since the Conway River.

Start an irregular descent to jump the upper Devils Ditch at 8.6 miles. ▶8 Mountain laurel shades the valley of upper Devils Ditch. The grassy trail is easy on your feet and lungs. Parallel the upper Devils Ditch to a road fork at 9.4 miles. Here, a roadbed leaves left to the Bearfence Mountain Shelter. Keep straight and meet the Appalachian Trail (AT) at 9.5 miles. ▶9 Turn right, northbound.

Ascend the AT through intertwined mountain laurel and squatty pines, gaining the southwest side of Bearfence Mountain. Switchback uphill among lichen-covered boulders, passing a rock on your

Conway River Loop Elevation Profile

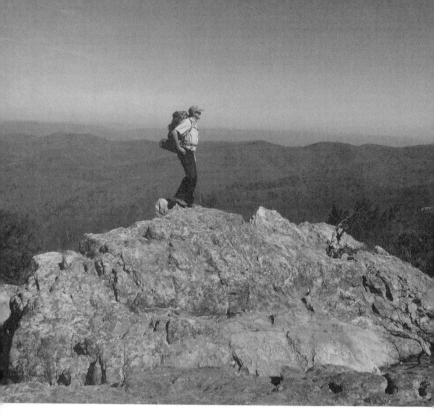

Crossing a view-laden perch *along the Bearfence Mountain Rock Scramble*

right that has views of Bluff Mountain to the east. Come to Bearfence Mountain Loop Trail at 10.1 miles. ►10 Turn right, taking the loop trail, and keep climbing. A short trail leads left to the obscure crest of Bearfence Mountain. Descend a bit and pass an outcrop on your left at 10.2 miles. ►11 It offers spectacular views of Skyline Drive, Massanutten Mountain, and the Shenandoah Valley below.

 Great Views

Come to the Bearfence Mountain Rock Scramble, marked with a concrete signpost, and turn right. The scramble is doable with a full backpack, but it is closed to pets. Carefully follow the blue blazes. Fantastic panoramas open in all directions, including the Conway River drainage from where you came. Fork Mountain, Jones Mountain, and Cat Knob rise across the Conway. This is one of the best views in

Mountain bellwort *graces the Conway River valley.*

Geological Interest

Ridgeline ▲

Wildflowers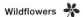

the park. Continue scrambling amid upthrust rocks with more views. Return to the AT at mile 10.6, and turn right. ▶12 It feels like a walk in the park. Skirt the edge of Bush Mountain beneath some large oak trees. A prolonged descent nears Skyline Drive. Slip over to the northeast side of the Blue Ridge. Wildflowers are abundant in spring here, from trillium to jack-in-the-pulpit. Reach Conway River Fire Road at mile 12.0. Take a few steps left on the fire road, and complete your loop. ▶13

🚶 MILESTONES

►1   0.0   Bootens Gap Parking Area at milepost 55.1

►2   1.4   Gate into Rapidan Wildlife Management Area

►3   2.6   Waterfall about 40 yards up a side stream

►4   3.8   Cross Conway River

►5   4.8   Cross Devils Ditch

►6   5.0   Cross Conway River

►7   5.5   Cross Conway River, and pick up Slaughter Trail

►8   8.6   Cross upper Devils Ditch

►9   9.5   Right on AT

►10   10.1   Right on Bearfence Mountain Loop Trail

►11   10.2   Enjoy view and then right at Bearfence Mountain Rock Scramble

►12   10.6   Right on AT

►13   12.0   Complete loop

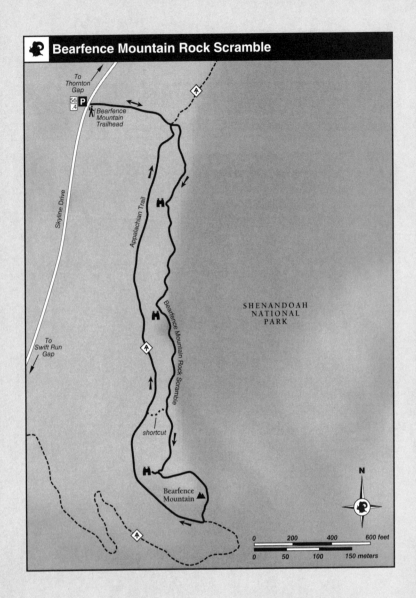

Bearfence Mountain Rock Scramble

To
Thornton
Gap

56
4 P

Bearfence
Mountain
Trailhead

Skyline Drive

To
Swift Run
Gap

Appalachian Trail

Bearfence Mountain Rock Scramble

shortcut

SHENANDOAH
NATIONAL
PARK

Bearfence
Mountain

N

0   200   400   600 feet
0   50   100   150 meters

Bearfence Mountain Rock Scramble

Best Time

Hike whenever the trails are dry and the sky is clear. The rocks will not be slippery then, and you can enjoy the first-rate panoramas beheld from atop Bearfence Mountain.

Finding the Trail

The hike starts at milepost 56.4 on Skyline Drive. From the Swift Run Gap Entrance Station, head north on Skyline Drive 9 miles to the Bearfence Mountain Parking Area, on your left.

Trail Description

The name Bearfence Mountain Rock Scramble is not only an intriguing moniker; it also conjures up images of scaling dangerous boulders on the side of a cliff. Yes, this is an exciting trek that requires the use of hands and feet in a few places, but it is neither dangerous nor difficult and can be done by all but the youngest and oldest of Shenandoah trail trekkers. Just go when the rock is dry, take your time, and be willing to give or ask for help from your fellow hikers if a spot or two seems tough, although one can easily execute the scramble without aid. For your efforts, you will find excellent views from open outcrops along this well-marked trail that combines with the Appalachian Trail (AT) to make a short but exhilarating loop.

Join the Bearfence Mountain Rock Scramble, a wide footpath at this point, leaving east from Skyline

TRAIL USE
Day Hiking,
Pets Prohibited
LENGTH
1.1 miles, 1–1.5 hours
VERTICAL FEET
±310
DIFFICULTY
– 1 2 **3** 4 5 +
TRAIL TYPE
Loop
START & FINISH
N38° 27.144'
W78° 28.014'

FEATURES
Ridgeline
Autumn Colors
Great Views
Geological Interest
FACILITIES
None

The view *from atop Bearfence Mountain*

Your climb rewards you with a Blue Ridge panorama.

Ridgeline ▲

Drive. ▶1 Quickly rise to intersect the AT at 0.1 mile. ▶2 Keep straight on the Bearfence Mountain Rock Scramble, still a standard foot trail. Wind your way through a mix of forest and emergent boulders, anticipating the scramble part of the trail. By 0.2 mile, you have opened onto a partial view atop an outcrop. When the trail joins the open rocky ridge and outcrops of Bearfence Mountain, the trail blazes—painted onto the outcrops themselves—are frequent, leading you amid crevices and stone faces,

Bearfence Mountain Rock Scramble Elevation Profile

where you will be using all fours in places. You may find yourself wondering where the trail will or should go next. At 0.3 mile, open onto an outcrop with 360-degree views of the Blue Ridge and lands falling away in all directions, one of the best panoramas in the Old Dominion. ►3 Continuing along the scramble, you may see the AT below you. At 0.4 mile, come to an intersection. Here a shortcut takes you right to the AT, but stay left, now on the Bearfence Loop Trail. The scrambling is over, but you do get to enjoy another view from a spur trail at 0.5 mile. The oak-framed vista, set on a rock outcrop, opens to the west. Massanutten Mountain and the Shenandoah Valley lie to the fore, and the ridges of West Virginia fade toward the setting sun (if you time it right).

Continue cruising Bearfence Mountain, passing a grassy potential picnic area, then dip to meet the AT at 0.6 mile. ►4 Turn right on the master path of Shenandoah National Park, northbound. Pass a noteworthy rock overhang to the left of the trail. Curve below the stony upthrusts of Bearfence Mountain, now in rocky woods. Walk upon laid-flat stones that resemble pavers. Pass the other end of the loop shortcut at 0.8 mile. Continue the downgrade, and you'll soon complete the loop portion of the hike at 1.0 mile. ►5 From here, it is but a short backtrack to the trailhead. ►6

Geological
Interest

Great Views

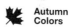
Autumn
Colors

	MILESTONES	
►1	0.0	Bearfence Mountain Rock Scramble parking
►2	0.1	Intersect Appalachian Trail
►3	0.3	Views in all directions, more views 0.1 mile ahead
►4	0.6	Right on Appalachian Trail
►5	1.0	Complete loop, left on Bearfence Mountain Rock Scramble
►6	1.1	Return to trailhead, completing the hike

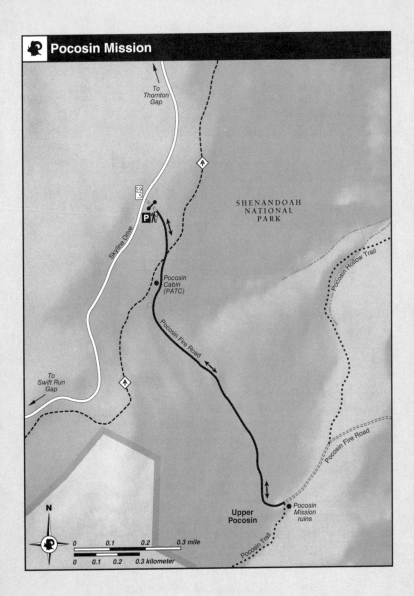

Pocosin Mission

To Thornton Gap

Skyline Drive

59 .5

P

SHENANDOAH
NATIONAL
PARK

Pocosin Hollow Trail

Pocosin Cabin
(PATC)

Pocosin Fire Road

To Swift Run Gap

Pocosin Fire Road

Upper
Pocosin

Pocosin
Mission
ruins

Pocosin Trail

N

| 0 | 0.1 | 0.2 | 0.3 mile |

| 0 | 0.1 | 0.2 | 0.3 kilometer |

Pocosin Mission

Take a walk into the past on this short trek. Leave Skyline Drive on the wide and easy Pocosin Fire Road, and explore the ruins of the Pocosin Mission, where a brave Episcopal minister attempted to save the souls of surrounding mountaineers. Explore the ruins of the mission and other nearby signs of habitation on a child-friendly walk. If you desire to walk a bit more, you can head down Pocosin Hollow. Descend to see many old-growth trees on your way down to a tumbling watercourse, where you'll find a nice spot to picnic or relax. Or you can take a stroll on an adjacent parcel of the Appalachian Trail (AT), and grab a view from a rocky slope.

Best Time

Because this hike is short, you can enjoy it at any time of year. In spring, however, you can view wildflowers and also better view the relics of the Pocosin Mission.

Finding the Trail

From Swift Run Gap, drive north on Skyline Drive for 6 miles to milepost 59.5. Look on your right for a road and a sign saying DO NOT BLOCK FIRE ROAD. Turn onto this road, and park in one of the gravel spots. The Pocosin Fire Road starts here. This road is 0.4 mile south of The Oaks Overlook and 1.6 miles north of Bald Face Mountain Overlook.

TRAIL USE
Day Hiking,
Child-Friendly

LENGTH
2.0 miles, 1–2 hours

VERTICAL FEET
±420

DIFFICULTY
– 1 **2** 3 4 5 +

TRAIL TYPE
Out-and-back

START & FINISH
N38° 24.798'
W78° 29.318'

FEATURES
Ridgeline
Autumn Colors
Wildflowers
Old-Growth Forest
Great Views
Historical Interest

FACILITIES
None

About Old-Growth Forests

Sometimes an old-growth forest isn't as evident as people expect. Before you imagine a continuous stand of giant trees, you must realize that authentic old-growth woodland is not an agglomeration of evenly aged trees. On the contrary, a forest made up of evenly aged trees is a sign of disturbance. An old-growth forest will have many big trees along with younger trees that grow when they get the chance. When a big tree falls, it creates a light gap. Young trees sprout in this light gap, and other already somewhat grown trees thrive in the additional sun. Trees are continually growing and dying, as older trees succumb to lightning strikes, disease, or old age, creating a mosaic of trees of all ages within an old-growth stand.

Trail Description

A lot of hikers miss this trailhead since it has a narrow entrance. After you find it, leave the parking area on the Pocosin Fire Road, a nearly level wide grade. ▶1 Intersect the AT at 0.1 mile. ▶2 A northern hardwood forest of red maple, sugar maple, basswood, and cherry rise overhead. Distinguishing between sugar maples and red maples is easy. Look at the leaf of a 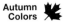 sugar maple. The curves between lobes of the sugar maple are U shaped, whereas the curves between lobes of the red maple are at right angles. Continue on the Pocosin Fire Road and come to a clearing at 0.2 mile. ▶3 This is the Pocosin Cabin, built in 1937

Autumn Colors

Pocosin Mission Elevation Profile

A hiker *checks out the ruins at the Pocosin Mission site.*

by the Civilian Conservation Corps. The Potomac Appalachian Trail Club (PATC), a philanthropic organization that maintains trails, rents this cabin to both its members and the general public.

The fire road drops moderately, still bordered by deciduous trees. The trail's width makes for easy hiking, and you soon pass a spring on trail left. It is used by AT hikers and those staying at the cabin. Come to a trail junction at 1.0 mile. ▶4 This spot is known as Upper Pocosin. To your right, through the trees, are the remnants of the Pocosin Mission.

Follow the footpath to the steps of the old church, built in 1904. Look at the walls made of native stone. The other nearby building is barely standing. Parts of the structure were built with hand-hewn logs; boards, nails, and even tar paper were later additions. Watch below you, as there is much broken glass, some parcels of clay pipe, and even pottery shards around. Look around also for the cemetery, where a few graves are marked with simple stones. As you tour the area, imagine

It's a short walk to these historic mission ruins.

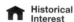 **Historical Interest**

the work of these missionaries, here in the remote Potomac Highlands, trying to spread Christianity among folk who had rarely traveled more than a day's horseback ride from home.

If you are looking for more trail mileage, head for Pocosin Hollow. To get there, continue down the Pocosin Fire Road, and veer left on the Pocosin Hollow Trail in a quarter mile. From this point forward, you should have the nut- and acorn-lined trail to yourself. Look for large old-growth trees scattered here and there along the path. The hike passes a boulder field before entering a wet draw, a rich wildflower area. Numerous old-growth yellow birch, oak, and tulip trees rise overhead. Reach the main watercourse of Pocosin Hollow, a tributary of the Conway River, 1.8 miles from the mission. A rock-hop takes you to the far side of the stream and a nice resting spot.

Another option is to backtrack from Pocosin Mission and meet the AT. For a decent view, head left, southbound, on the AT. You travel through rocky woods on a singletrack path, passing a spur to the PATC cabin. Climb rocky steps, winding through boulders on an artistically constructed trail leading to an outcrop with an easterly view a quarter mile from the Pocosin Fire Road. Even if you don't add these side hikes to the Pocosin Mission trek, you will be well rewarded.

Old-Growth Forest

Wildflowers

Ridgeline

Great Views

🚶 MILESTONES

►1	0.0	Pocosin Fire Road Parking Area at milepost 59.5
►2	0.1	Cross Appalachian Trail
►3	0.2	PATC Pocosin Cabin
►4	1.0	Trail intersection and Pocosin Mission

South River Falls Loop

Gravity plays a big role in this hike. Make an easy descent, and see South River Falls drop 80 feet over a rock face from a perched vista. Go farther and enjoy the view from the base of the falls. You'll have to fight the earth's tug on your climb out of the South River watershed and back to the former mountaintop pastureland, but the falls are worth the climb. This is a rich wildflower area in spring.

Best Time

Winter and spring see South River Falls at their boldest. In addition, spring wildflowers are rich in this valley. Summer offers cool deep woods. Autumn colors are worthy, but the falls flow less vigorously.

Finding the Trail

The trailhead is at the South River Picnic Ground, at milepost 62.8 on Skyline Drive. The path starts at the back of the picnic area on the one-way loop road. The trailhead is on your right. The picnic area entrance is 2.7 miles north of the Swift Run Gap Entrance Station on Skyline Drive.

Trail Description

Leave the rear of the pleasant South River Picnic Ground on a wide dirt footpath, ▶1 the South River Falls Trail, and intersect the Appalachian Trail (AT). Watch for piled rocks in this long-ago-overgrown farmland. Continue down to a switchback at 0.4 mile.

TRAIL USE
Day Hiking

LENGTH
4.5 miles, 2–3 hours

VERTICAL FEET
±1,000'

DIFFICULTY
− 1 2 **3** 4 5 +

TRAIL TYPE
Loop

START & FINISH
N38° 22.860'
W78° 31.021'

FEATURES
Stream
Waterfall
Autumn Colors
Wildflowers
Geological Interest

FACILITIES
Picnic tables
Restroom
Water

FLORA

Yellow Birches

Yellow birch trees shade mossy rocks and ferns. Look for peeling yellowish-gold bark with horizontal stripes. Larger yellow birches peel on their upper branches, not on their lower trunks. The twigs and leaves, when crushed, have a slight wintergreen aroma. Primarily a tree of the north ranging from Minnesota to Maine, yellow birches stretch down the spine of the Appalachians all the way to the South Carolina and Georgia mountain regions. They can be found in moist, cool environments throughout the mountains of Virginia.

Yellow birches often sprout on nutrient-rich rotting logs. Later, the yellow birch grows and the log rots completely away, leaving the yellow birch to look as if it grew legs.

▶2 Twist and turn three more times before coming to the South River, which is a small but wide creek at this point. Cross a side branch and enjoy the lush streamside environment.

Violets, toothwort, white trillium, and wild geranium color the moist margins, as do straight-trunked tulip trees and gray beeches. Other wildflowers include trout lily, false Solomon's seal, jack-in-the-pulpit, and columbine. Come to a second tributary at 0.7 mile. The valley narrows, and so does the stream. Cross a rock field at 1.0 mile, then step across a boulder-strewn tributary. Ahead and to your right is the top of the falls, but keep going—there's a better and safer viewpoint a short distance past the granite overhang to your left. Walk out on the outcrop, bordered with a man-made stone wall to your right and see South River Falls. ▶3 It spills over a rock face and then splits into two chutes charging downward. There is so much more light here than in the dark streamside environment. South River Falls is spotlighted as well.

The South River is slowly, unceasingly cutting into the precipitous stone barricade. Saddleback Mountain rises to your left. To get a different

 Stream

 Wildflowers

This trip is one of the park's better wildflower destinations.

 Geological Interest

 Waterfall

South River Falls *splits into channels as it drops.*

Wildflowers

perspective continue down the trail, reaching a junction at 1.4 miles. Veer right toward the base of the falls. ▶4 Curve past a tributary into a fertile wildflower zone. Notice the boundary with the Rapidan Wildlife Management Area, a State of Virginia property bordering the park. Descend to river level again and reach a flat. Head upriver on a narrow foot trail, passing an impressive fractured rock rampart to your right. Stone steps aid your ascent. Come to the

South River Falls Loop Elevation Profile

base of South River Falls at 2.1 miles. ▶5 Looking up, you can clearly see the narrow chute splitting in two before resuming a calmer path toward the sea. This view is superior to the higher falls perspective.

Waterfall

Finish your uphill backtracking at 2.8 miles, then veer right onto new trail, rising toward the South River Fire Road. ▶6 You can still hear the roar of South River Falls. Meet the South River Fire Road at 3.2 miles. ▶7 Turn left and continue a moderate ascent on a wide track. A lucky hiker might see yellow lady slippers hereabouts in season. Meet the AT at 4.1 miles. ▶8 Turn left here, southbound, traveling through younger woods mixed with pine on a singletrack path. Complete the loop portion of the hike at 4.4 miles. Turn right on the South River Falls Trail to reach the South River Picnic Ground. ▶9 Enjoy a well-deserved lunch or cookout after your hiking adventure.

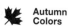

Autumn Colors

	MILESTONES	
▶1	0.0	South River Picnic Ground
▶2	0.4	First switchback
▶3	1.3	Upper observation point of South River Falls
▶4	1.4	Right turn toward base of falls
▶5	2.1	Base of South River Falls
▶6	2.8	Veer right toward South River Fire Road
▶7	3.2	Left on South River Fire Road
▶8	4.1	Left, southbound, on the AT
▶9	4.5	Return to South River Picnic Ground

CHAPTER 3

South District

South District

The South District is the least visited of the park's three districts. Partly because it is more distant from the Washington metroplex, the South District has a more relaxed, remote aura. It also has the fewest visitor facilities, which are limited to the Loft Mountain area, with a camp store and campground, and Dundo Picnic Ground, a few miles south of Loft Mountain. US 33 connecting Elkton to Stanardsville marks the north end of the South District. The district stretches south to Rockfish Gap near Waynesboro, connected by 40 miles of Skyline Drive.

The South District has many characteristics that separate it from the others. First, it has the largest acreage of designated wilderness. It also is the lowest in elevation but is the rockiest parcel of this boulder-laden park. It has the park's biggest stream—Big Run. The trails here are the least hiked, especially if you get off the Appalachian Trail (AT).

Hiking opportunities are numerous and varied in length, difficulty, and destination. Heading south from Swift Run Gap, you can first hike to Hightop, where a wildflower-bordered track rises to outcrops with westerly vistas limited only by the clarity of the sky. Both Rocky Mount and Rocky Mountain are quartz-tipped mountain crests divided by steep drainages where translucent streams gurgle through wild corridors. They offer secluded trekking experiences.

Enjoy more views from Loft Mountain, as well as human history and the convenience of incorporating park facilities into a hike. Saunter among the pines on Patterson Ridge on a challenging loop that travels high and low. Big Run Loop takes you from Skyline Drive to the upper Big Run watershed before using the AT to close the loop.

Rockytop Mountain not only recalls the University of Tennessee fight song of the same name but also lives up to its name. Incredible and nearly continuous views characterize this fire-scarred, stone-pocked ridge. Lower Big Run is a wild stream with big pools, rapids, and plenty of room to roam. Austin Mountain is another rocky crest that is peppered with

Opposite and overleaf: *A boulder field provides an excellent view from atop Turk Mountain (Trail 50, page 321).*

221

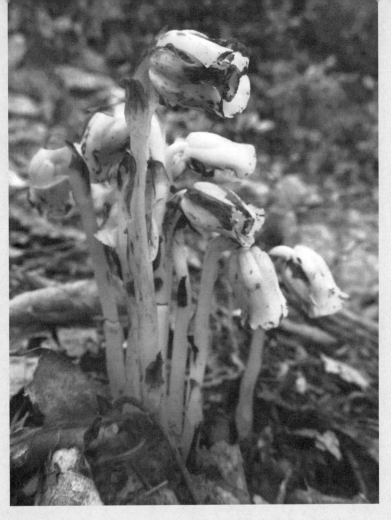

Indian ghost pipe *emerges from the summer forest floor.*

evergreens and laden with views of the surrounding terrain in a solitude unimagined elsewhere in the park. The Falls Loop from Browns Gap drops off the east side of the Blue Ridge and makes a circuit along two waterfall-rich streams in Doyles River and Jones Run. Old-growth trees on Jones Run are an added treat.

Furnace Mountain is one of those hidden gems passed over by most hikers. Conversely, Blackrock, a geological wonder, is a popular peak that presents spectacular landscapes from its boulder garden summit. Farther south, Moormans River marks distant terrain, with Big Branch Falls a highlight. Hikers can access Chimney Rock, with its first-rate views from either Riprap Hollow, where falls and pools ease a climb, or from Skyline Drive, where you travel rocky terrain from the AT, running the spine of South District.

Turk Mountain is one peak almost everyone can bag. And the vistas from there are simply stunning. Put together, the hikes here, whether loops or out-and-backs, present the best of the South District.

Permits

Permits are not required for day hiking. Backpackers must get a backcountry permit to stay in the backcountry. Simple self-registration stations are located at Swift Run Gap Entrance Station, Loft Mountain Wayside, and Rockfish Gap Entrance Station.

Maps

For the South District, here are the relevant U.S. Geological Survey 7.5-minute (1:24,000-scale) topographic quadrangles, listed in geographic order as you hike along your route:

Trail 34: *Swift Run Gap*
Trail 35: *McGaheysville*
Trail 36: *McGaheysville*
Trail 37: *McGaheysville*
Trail 38: *McGaheysville*
Trail 39: *McGaheysville* and *Browns Cove*
Trail 40: *Browns Cove* and *McGaheysville*
Trail 41: *Browns Cove, McGaheysville,* and *Grottoes*
Trail 42: *Browns Cove*
Trail 43: *Browns Cove, McGaheysville, Grottoes,* and *Crimora*
Trail 44: *Browns Cove* and *Crimora*
Trail 45: *Browns Cove*
Trail 46: *Browns Cove*
Trail 47: *Crimora, Browns Cove,* and *Waynesboro East*
Trail 48: *Crimora*
Trail 49: *Crimora*
Trail 50: *Crimora* and *Waynesboro East*

South District

McGaheysville

Swift Run Gap
Entrance Station

To
Stanardsville

Hightop

34

Longs
Hill

Rocky
Mount

Skyline Drive

Shenandoah River

35

36

Grottoes

Rockytop

37 38

Loft
Mountain

SHENANDOAH
NATIONAL
PARK

Austin
Mountain

39

Loft Mountain
Campground

40 41 42

Big Flat
Mountain

43

Trayfoot
Mountain

44 45

Cedar
Mountain

Skyline Drive

46

Cherry
Mountain

Rocks
Mountain

47 48 49

Pasture Fence
Mountain

Crimora

Pigeon Top
Mountain

50

Bucks Elbow
Mountain

Ramsey
Mountain

Calf
Mountain

Crozet

Turners
Mountain

Waynesboro

N

Scott
Mountain

Greenwood

Rockfish Gap
Entrance Station

Skyline Drive

84

To
Charlottesville

250

0   1   2   3 miles

0 1 2 3 kilometers

TRAIL FEATURES TABLE

South District

TRAIL	Difficulty	Length	Type	USES & ACCESS	TERRAIN	NATURE	OTHER
34	3	3.2	Out-and-Back	Day Hiking, Backpacking	Summit	Autumn Colors, Wildflowers	Great Views, Geological Interest
35	5	9.8	Loop	Day Hiking, Backpacking	Summit, Ridgeline, Stream	Autumn Colors, Wildflowers	Great Views, Historical Interest, Geological Interest
36	5	9.5	Loop	Day Hiking, Backpacking	Ridgeline, Stream, Waterfall	Autumn Colors	Great Views, Swimming, Steep, Geological Interest
37	2	2.9	Out-and-Back	Day Hiking, Pets Prohibited	Ridgeline	Autumn Colors, Wildflowers	Great Views, Camping, Geological Interest
38	5	9.7	Loop	Day Hiking, Backpacking	Ridgeline, Stream	Autumn Colors	Great Views, Camping, Swimming, Secluded
39	3	5.8	Loop	Day Hiking	Ridgeline, Stream	Autumn Colors, Wildflowers	Great Views, Historical Interest, Geological Interest
40	5	13.3	Loop	Day Hiking, Backpacking	Ridgeline, Stream	Autumn Colors	Great Views, Swimming, Secluded, Steep, Historical Interest
41	4	8.8	Loop	Day Hiking, Backpacking	Ridgeline, Stream	Autumn Colors, Wildflowers	Great Views, Historical Interest
42	4	7.0	Loop	Day Hiking, Backpacking	Ridgeline, Stream, Waterfall	Autumn Colors, Wildflowers, Old-Growth Forest	Historical Interest, Geological Interest
43	5	20.7	Loop	Day Hiking, Backpacking	Summit, Ridgeline, Stream	Autumn Colors, Wildflowers, Wildlife	Great Views, Swimming, Secluded, Historical Interest, Geological Interest
44	3	6.8	Out-and-Back	Day Hiking, Backpacking	Summit	Autumn Colors	Great Views, Secluded, Geological Interest
45	1	1.1	Loop	Day Hiking, Child-Friendly	Summit, Ridgeline	Autumn Colors	Great Views, Geological Interest
46	4	7.6	Out-and-Back	Day Hiking, Backpacking	Stream, Waterfall	Autumn Colors, Wildflowers	Swimming, Secluded
47	5	18.3	Loop	Day Hiking, Backpacking	Ridgeline, Stream, Waterfall	Autumn Colors, Wildflowers, Wildlife	Great Views, Swimming, Secluded, Historical Interest
48	2	3.2	Out-and-Back	Day Hiking, Backpacking	Ridgeline	Autumn Colors	Great Views, Geological Interest
49	4	7.5	Loop	Day Hiking, Backpacking	Ridgeline, Stream, Waterfall	Autumn Colors, Wildflowers	Secluded, Historical Interest
50	2	2.4	Out-and-Back	Day Hiking	Summit, Ridgeline	Autumn Colors	Great Views, Secluded, Geological Interest

Legend

TYPE
- Loop
- Out-and-Back
- DIFFICULTY − 1 2 3 4 5 + (less … more)

USES & ACCESS
- Day Hiking
- Backpacking
- Child-Friendly
- Pets Prohibited

TERRAIN
- Summit
- Ridgeline
- Stream
- Waterfall

NATURE
- Autumn Colors
- Wildflowers
- Wildlife
- Old-Growth Forest

FEATURES
- Great Views
- Camping
- Swimming
- Secluded
- Steep
- Historical Interest
- Geological Interest

South District

Patterson Ridge Loop 251

This tough loop unites a remote wilderness trail, the park's biggest stream, some high country, and a campground. The infrequently hiked Patterson Ridge Trail descends to Big Run. Rock-hop your way along the watercourse, then climb to Skyline Drive. Join the fabled Appalachian Trail, heading northbound passing near Loft Mountain Campground.

TRAIL 38

Day Hiking,
Backpacking
9.7 miles, Loop
Difficulty: 1 2 3 4 **5**

Big Run Loop 257

Explore several types of forest and mountain lands. Leave Big Run Overlook, and head into prototype oak woods. Travel a dry piney ridgeline with its attendant mountain laurel. Make your way to a moist valley harboring cove hardwoods. Join the Appalachian Trail and the spine of the Blue Ridge, hiking amid boulder fields and bluffs.

TRAIL 39

Day Hiking
5.8 miles, Loop
Difficulty: 1 2 **3** 4 5

Rockytop and Big Run Loop 263

Ramble the high ridge of Rockytop Mountain where talus slopes and open boulders make for solitude-filled lookouts of the adjacent mountainscape and Shenandoah Valley beyond. Drop into crystalline Big Run, exploring the gorgeous valley of the park's largest watershed from low to high.

TRAIL 40

Day Hiking,
Backpacking
13.3 miles, Loop
Difficulty: 1 2 3 4 **5**

Austin Mountain and Madison Run Loop 269

Leave historic Browns Gap, tracing a modernized toll path, joining Austin Mountain Trail. Hike past clearings and over several talus slopes, availing seldom-seen outstanding views. Descend in pines to Madison Run, where rich forest shades a trout stream. Trek up the valley, winding along ridges and hollows back to Browns Gap.

TRAIL 41

Day Hiking,
Backpacking
8.8 miles, Loop
Difficulty: 1 2 3 **4** 5

TRAIL 42

Day Hiking,
Backpacking
7.0 miles, Loop
Difficulty: 1 2 3 **4** 5

Falls Loop from Browns Gap 275

Water lovers will fall for this loop. The trail passes three major cataracts and numerous other cascades as it explores two boulder-strewn canyons connected by the Appalachian Trail. The hike up Jones Run passes some old-growth tulip trees with impressive girths.

TRAIL 43

Day Hiking,
Backpacking
20.7 miles, Loop
Difficulty: 1 2 3 4 **5**

Trayfoot Mountain Loop 279

This backpacking circuit combines the Appalachian Trail, remote rock ridges, and mountain streams with multiple panoramas from multiple locations, allowing you to see where you are going and where you were. The hike's challenges are felt in two major climbs.

TRAIL 44

Day Hiking,
Backpacking
6.8 miles, Out-and-back
Difficulty: 1 2 **3** 4 5

Furnace Mountain via Blackrock ... 287

This geologically rich hike visits huge outcrops and open talus slopes where rocks by the thousands carpet the mountainsides. You'll first soak in the outstanding views of Blackrock Summit with plenty of company, then a rocky trail leads to the solitude of Furnace Mountain and a fine vista.

TRAIL 45

Day Hiking,
Child-Friendly
1.1 miles, Loop
Difficulty: **1** 2 3 4 5

Blackrock Loop 293

Start at nearly 3,000 feet, and hike to an incredible rock jumble on the Appalachian Trail. Views extend for miles in multiple directions from the summit of Blackrock. After gaining views from several spots, reenter woods, and work your way back to the trailhead.

Big Branch Falls via Moormans River 297

This trail-accessible waterfall is seldom reached from Skyline Drive, despite being a scenic route. First, descend to the North Fork Moormans River, with cascades and pools in a deep valley bordered by high ridges. Finally, climb along low-flow Big Branch, with its open watery bowls divided by rock slabs where the stream falls in slide cascades.

TRAIL 46

Day Hiking,
Backpacking
7.6 miles, Out-and-back
Difficulty: 1 2 3 **4** 5

Moormans River Loop 301

This long circuit first leads atop the Blue Ridge before dropping into the upper Moormans River watershed, where you walk along both scenic forks of the Moormans River before regaining the Blue Ridge. Highlights include Shenandoah panoramas, and the North Fork Moormans River valley with its big pools. The South Fork Moormans River reveals more cascades and serene pools that attract bathers in summer.

TRAIL 47

Day Hiking,
Backpacking
18.3 miles, Loop
Difficulty: 1 2 3 4 **5**

Chimney Rock 309

Take the Appalachian Trail under oaks to rocky Riprap Trail. Cruise past a stony vista, and then hike past boulder gardens to reach Chimney Rock, a distended stone spire presenting views of the adjacent talus-covered peaks and Shenandoah Valley beyond.

TRAIL 48

Day Hiking,
Backpacking
3.2 miles, Out-and-back
Difficulty: 1 **2** 3 4 5

Turk Branch Loop 315

Leave the crest of the Blue Ridge and descend along remote Turk Branch. Head up the uppermost part of the rocky South Fork Moormans River valley to meet the Appalachian Trail. Hike north on Shenandoah's master path, gaining limited views amid the pines and oaks before returning to Turk Gap. Though the elevation change is nearly 1,200 feet, the trail grades are never sharp.

TRAIL 49

Day Hiking,
Backpacking
7.5 miles, Loop
Difficulty: 1 2 3 **4** 5

TRAIL 50

Day Hiking
2.4 miles, Out-and-back
Difficulty: 1 **2** 3 4 5

Turk Mountain 321

Hike to a boulder-strewn summit. This dead-end trek rises from quiet Turk Gap. Wander woodland to emerge at the crest of Turk Mountain, where a huge talus slope opens the sky to limitless western vistas of Shenandoah Valley.

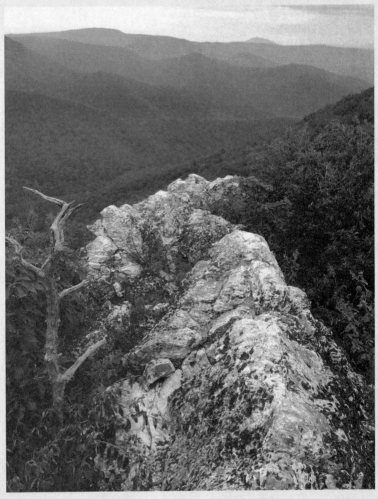

Gazing into the Big Run valley *from one of the many outcrops atop aptly named Rocky Mountain (Trail 36, page 241)*

Hightop

This is one peak that almost everyone can bag. Just at the point where novice hikers get tired of climbing, the path tops out and presents a very rewarding view. Get a taste of the Appalachian Trail (AT) while climbing one of the park's higher mountains.

Best Time

Fall through spring is optimal for this hike. You can enjoy wildflowers and far-reaching views in spring. Summer can be hazy. Fall has colors and clarity of sky. Winter offers clear days and sure solitude.

Finding the Trail

The Hightop Mountain Parking Area is located at milepost 66.7 on Skyline Drive. From the Swift Run Gap Entrance Station, drive south on Skyline Drive for 1.2 miles to the parking area on your right.

Trail Description

Start the trek by crossing Skyline Drive from the Hightop Mountain Parking Area. ▶1 Pick up the AT, southbound. Hike through a bramble- and briar-covered area on a moderate uphill grade. This area is transitioning from field to forest. Enter woods and pass two large gray boulders acting as sentinels for the mountaintop ahead. Ahead, more lichen-covered boulders line the path, which becomes rocky as it climbs. The adjacent woods can be rocky too. Step over a gurgling spring branch that runs dry by fall. Cross an older and

TRAIL USE
Day Hiking,
Backpacking

LENGTH
3.2 miles, 2–3 hours

VERTICAL FEET
±950'

DIFFICULTY
– 1 2 **3** 4 5 +

TRAIL TYPE
Out-and-back

START & FINISH
N38° 20.713'
W78° 33.178'

FEATURES
Summit
Autumn Colors
Wildflowers
Great Views
Geological Interest

FACILITIES
None

 Geological Interest

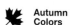 **Autumn Colors**

231

Hightop

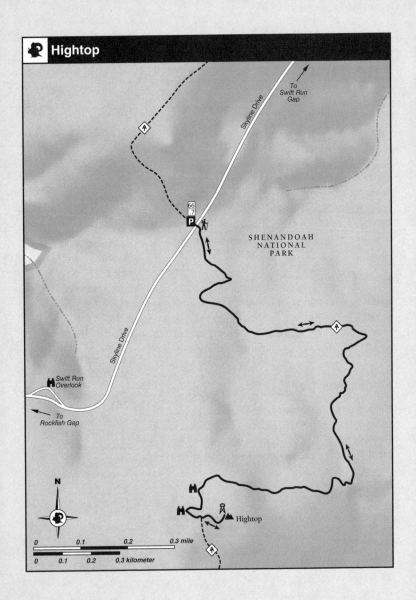

To
Swift Run
Gap

Skyline Drive

66
.7

P

SHENANDOAH
NATIONAL
PARK

Skyline Drive

Swift Run
Overlook

To
Rockfish Gap

N

Hightop

| 0 | 0.1 | 0.2 | 0.3 mile |
| 0 | 0.1 | 0.2 | 0.3 kilometer |

steeper trail at 0.5 mile—good thing that way to the top was abandoned. ▶2 This side of Hightop is a rich wildflower area in spring. Expect to see white trillium, as well as the overhanging maroon blooms of Catesby's trillium. Other wildflowers you may see include wild geranium, mayapples, and star chickweed. A level section ahead offers a brief reprieve before the AT starts switchbacking up the mountain at a steeper grade. At mile 1.0, the trail again levels, this time in a gap. ▶3 The larger oak and tulip trees at this elevation take on a gnarled appearance; the weather can be rough up here and the trees show it. But nature has a gentler side on Hightop too that is evident by its verdant fertility in early spring (May and early June).

 Wildflowers

The AT swings around the right side of Hightop, soon passing two outcrops that offer first-rate vistas. The first outcrop, at 1.4 miles, reveals Massanutten Peak straight ahead. ▶4 To your right is the town of Elkton, and of course, the Shenandoah Valley stretches out below. North Mountain is in the farthest distance and can be seen on clear days. The cluster of houses just below is the community of Sandy Bottom.

 Great Views

The next outcrop, also to the right of the trail, is clearly more spectacular and a just reward for your efforts. ▶5 The rock face of Rocky Mount stands

Hightop Elevation Profile

Great Views 🔭

plainly visible. The bulk of Shenandoah's mountains extend in wave upon wave in the distance. The mass to your left is Flattop Mountain. Skyline Drive flows just below you.

Continue a short distance farther until you come to a trace of a trail leading left. A concrete signpost indicates the AT leaving right and downhill for Hightop trail hut, then on down to Georgia. Consider visiting the hut if you want to add 1.2 miles to your hike. Follow the trail left and quickly get to the level top of Hightop, at 3,587 feet, at mile 1.6. ▶6 Views are limited here since the fire tower was dismantled, but it makes a good lunch spot if the winds are high or the sun excessively strong on the outcrops. From the trailhead, you gained nearly 1,000 feet of altitude in less than 2 miles.

Summit ⛰️

🚶	MILESTONES	
▶1	0.0	Hightop Parking Area at milepost 66.7
▶2	0.5	Old steep track crosses the AT
▶3	1.0	Gap
▶4	1.4	First outcrop with views
▶5	1.5	Second outcrop with spectacular views
▶6	1.6	Left at short trail to Hightop Peak

Rocky Mount Loop

If you like wilderness hiking in solitude, take this ambitious loop. Leave the main crest of the Blue Ridge to access the summit of Rocky Mount for far-reaching views. Descend sharply to Gap Run and return up the watershed to the Rocky Mount Trail. You'll have this untamed slice of Shenandoah to yourself.

Best Time

You will experience solitude just about any time of year. Spring offers extensive views, as well as wildflowers along Gap Run. Summer can be hazy and sometimes warm. Fall sports colors and clear skies again. Winter is a good time too, especially after fronts, when the air is crisp and clear.

Finding the Trail

The trailhead can be found 0.1 mile north of Two Mile Run Overlook, at milepost 76.2 on Skyline Drive. It is 10.7 miles south of the Swift Run Gap Entrance Station, on the west side of Skyline Drive.

Trail Description

You may see evidence such as scarred tree trunks from the April 2016 Rocky Mount Fire—the second largest fire in park history—which burned more than 10,000 acres in the area before it was contained. This area of the park hadn't seen fire in 85 years, so the conflagration should have positive effects on forest health in the Rocky Mount area.

TRAIL USE
Day Hiking,
Backpacking
LENGTH
9.8 miles, 6–7 hours
VERTICAL FEET
±2,200'
DIFFICULTY
– 1 2 3 4 **5** +
TRAIL TYPE
Loop
START & FINISH
N38° 17.942'
W78° 38.821'

FEATURES
Summit
Ridgeline
Stream
Autumn Colors
Wildflowers
Great Views
Historical Interest
Geological Interest

FACILITIES
None

Rocky Mount Loop

SHENANDOAH
NATIONAL
PARK

Rocky Mount Trail

▲ Rocky Mount

Gap Run Trail

Gap Run

Two Mile Run

Hawksbill Creek

628

To
Swift Run
Gap

Skyline Drive

Beldor Hollow
Overlook

One Mile Run

One Mile Run Trail

Rocky Mount Trail

Two Mile Run
Overlook

76
2

(No parking
at trailhead)

Brown Mountain Trail

Brown
Mountain
Overlook

To
Rockfish
Gap

Skyline Drive

Pinefield
Gap

N

0   0.2   0.4   0.6 mile

0   0.2 0.4 0.6 kilometer

Be careful walking along Skyline Drive to the trail's beginning. ▶1 Rocky Mount Trail starts at the north end of the rock wall stretching from Two Mile Run Overlook. Immediately climb a wooded knoll before dropping northeast on a narrow ridge. The lightly used singletrack foot trail alternately dips and levels off in oak-dominated woods before coming to a saddle at 0.7 mile. Veer to the left, southwest, side of the ridge among pine woods. To your left are intermittent views of Rocky Mountain (not to be confused with Rocky Mount) between scads of mountain laurel. You can also possibly look back at your car at Two Mile Run Overlook.

▲ Ridgeline

At 1.1 miles, come to a gap, ▶2 then swing around the northeast end of an unnamed knob. The valley of Hawksbill Creek drops far below. The forest changes to birch trees with a high canopy. Descend to rejoin the ridgecrest at 1.6 miles. Continue downhill. Rocky Mount lurks ever higher through the trees ahead. Reach another gap and a trail junction at 2.2 miles. ▶3 To the right is Gap Run Trail, your return route.

Continue straight on Rocky Mount Trail, beginning your 800-foot climb up the south face of Rocky Mount. Look between the oaks, pines, and azaleas lining the path back at Two Mile Run Overlook. The hollow of Two Mile Run lies below. Cross a partly forested talus slope at 2.6 miles and then switchback.

Rocky Mount Loop Elevation Profile

Looking back *to Two Mile Run Overlook from the top of Rocky Mount*

Geological Interest �",

Twice you think you're nearing the summit, but the stony trail keeps snaking through rocks and boulders.

Come to a side trail on your left just before reaching the true top of Rocky Mount at 3.3 miles. ▶4 It leads to a pine-framed outcrop with stunning views. A white quartz wall runs to your left. Look out over Two Mile Run. At the head of the run stands Two Mile Run Overlook, where you started, and the crest of the Blue Ridge. One Mile Run cuts the next valley south. Rocky Mountain rises beyond that. To your right stretches the South Fork Shenandoah River and the farms and fields that surround it.

Great Views 👀

Stream 🏞

Climb a bit, then reach the wooded peak of Rocky Mount (2,741'). The now lesser-used trail drops along the base of a huge granite slope. Continue descending through a heavily canopied forest before coming to a pine stand with views into Gap Run. On a switchback, the rocky slope of Beldor Ridge is visible directly ahead. Traverse a rock field at mile 4.4, and reach a tributary of Gap Run at 4.6 miles. ▶5 Rock-hop the streamlet, dotted with pale rocks, twice in succession. Make a sharp right turn into a clearing before reaching Gap Run at 5.3 miles. ▶6 This is an easy rock-hop during normal flows. A concrete signpost stands on the far side of the creek. It is 0.7 mile downstream to the park boundary.

Stream 🏞

Turn right on Gap Run Trail, gently ascending an old road that has been washed out in places. Look for black birch shading this cooler, moister vale. Backpackers find legal campsites in the flats of Gap Run. Pass a clearing, once a homesite, worth exploring, and come to a second signpost at mile 5.5.

Historical Interest

Stay on the roadbed, and enter the rock-strewn flood plain of Gap Run. Overflow channels braid the woods, leaving the exact path unclear. Look for blue paint blazes marking the trail, and pick up the roadbed again, coming to another trail signpost at mile 6.0. ▶7 An old road leaves the park left. Dogwoods and white pines are sprinkled throughout the young forest, which was a field when this park was established. Turn right and travel along Gap Run, crossing the creek and its tributaries easily.

Wildflowers

Stream

Cross Gap Run a final time at 7.2 miles. ▶8 The trail grade sharpens, and Gap Run Trail follows a stony, dry wash toward a low spot on Rocky Mount Trail. Leave the dry wash at a switchback, and surge upward a short distance, reaching the gap at 7.6 miles. ▶9 You were here before. Turn left on Rocky Mount Trail, and retrace your steps 2.2 miles back to Skyline Drive and the Blue Ridge. ▶10

🚶	**MILESTONES**	
▶1	0.0	Two Mile Run Overlook at milepost 76.2
▶2	1.1	Gap
▶3	2.2	At gap and Gap Run Trail, stay left on Rocky Mount Trail
▶4	3.3	Vista and then summit of Rocky Mount
▶5	4.6	Tributary of Gap Run
▶6	5.3	Reach and cross Gap Run
▶7	6.0	Old road leaves left at post; Gap Run Trail stays right
▶8	7.2	Cross Gap Run a final time
▶9	7.6	At end of Gap Run Trail, stay left on Rocky Mount Trail
▶10	9.8	Two Mile Run Overlook at milepost 76.2

Rocky Mountain Loop

Two Mile Run

Two Mile Run Overlook

To Swift Run Gap

One Mile Run

Skyline Drive

Brown Mountain Trail

Brown Mountain Overlook

Ivy Creek Overlook

SHENANDOAH NATIONAL PARK

Brown Mountain Trail

Rockytop Overlook

Skyline Drive

To Rockfish Gap

Rocky Mountain Run Trail

Rocky Mountain Run

N

0.6 mile

0.4

0.6 kilometer

0.2

0.4

0.2

0

Patterson Ridge Trail

Big Run Portal Trail

Big Run

Big Run Portal Trail

Rocky Mountain Loop

This challenging hike entails a lot of ups and downs; the loop explores varied natural environments enhanced with copious vistas. Bring your camera. Take the Brown Mountain Trail, passing over Rocky Mountain and scenery reminiscent of the West, with stone spires rising from the forest before ending up at the park's largest watercourse, Big Run. Follow Big Run and Rocky Mountain Run back to the high country. Note that the first half of this hike is dry and that fording Big Run can be hazardous in high water.

In the South District, you have Rockytop, Rocky Mount, and Rocky Mountain all adjacent to one another. The names can be confusing, but each ridgeline presents distinct and scenic hiking opportunities. On this hike you are on Rocky Mountain, yet looking out on Rocky Mount and Rockytop.

Best Time

This loop requires crossing unbridged Big Run and Rocky Mountain Run numerous times, so it is best done when the streams are lower—late spring through late fall—and before the chills of winter make stream crossings numbing. Try to time your hikes after fronts clear the skies for views from Rocky Mountain and Brown Mountain. However, summer is best for splashing in the waters of Big Run.

Finding the Trail

The hike starts at the center of Brown Mountain Overlook at milepost 76.9 on Skyline Drive.

TRAIL USE
Day Hiking,
Backpacking

LENGTH
9.5 miles, 6–7.5 hours

VERTICAL FEET
±1,580'

DIFFICULTY
– 1 2 3 4 **5** +

TRAIL TYPE
Loop

START & FINISH
N38° 17.543'
W78° 39.480'

FEATURES
Ridgeline
Stream
Waterfall
Autumn Colors
Great Views
Swimming
Steep
Geological Interest

FACILITIES
None

Trail Description

Leave Brown Mountain Overlook behind, ►1 and steeply descend through a low clearing that opens to Rocky Mountain across the gap to your west and Big Run below. Rocky Mount stands to the north, and Rockytop forms a wall to the south. Leave the low-slung sumac and locust at 0.1 mile, entering full-blown hardwoods. The track switchbacks a narrow ridgeline to reach a gap and trail junction at 0.6 mile. ►2 To your left is the terminus of the Rocky Mountain Run Trail, your return route.

Continue straight on the Brown Mountain Trail, climbing the eastern flank of Rocky Mountain amid chestnut oaks. Achieve the ridgetop via switchbacks at 1.0 mile, passing through pines. The trail begins undulating along the stony spine of Rocky Mountain, emerging at a giant quartz outcrop at 1.5 miles. ►3 You can plainly see the crest of the Blue Ridge and Brown Mountain Overlook across the gulf of Rocky Mountain Run. Below, Big Run falls deeply beneath. Waves of mountains roll southward. This vista could be a rewarding 3-mile, out-and-back endeavor if the whole loop is too ambitious.

Beyond the outcrop, the stony track descends along the north side of Rocky Mountain under oaks, black gum, and hickory. At 2.5 miles, the now-sandy trail enters scattered pines standing over the

Ridgeline

Great Views

Autumn Colors

Rocky Mountain Loop Elevation Profile

low brush of blueberries. Views open. Massanutten Peak is dead ahead. Continue along the ridge, and top out on wooded Brown Mountain at mile 3.2.

Prepare for some of the finest scenery in Shenandoah National Park. Begin an irregular descent with many vistas. You'll have trouble keeping your balance on this rock-strewn trail as it switchbacks among pine and mountain laurel down the face of Brown Mountain. Why? There are multiple distracting views: Rocky Mountain, Rockytop, Big Run, Massanutten Peak, and Shenandoah Valley. Short spur trails lead to pine-framed outcrops and these views. At 3.5 miles, the trail regains the crest of the ridge. At 3.7 miles, hike downhill into a slope of patchy pines surviving between rock slabs. ►4 Here, gaze across Bearwallow Hollow at great stone protuberances on the far ridge. At 4.1 miles, the path curves into Big Run valley. The dry westfacing slope of sporadic pines, oaks, and blueberries affords views of white columnar spires, and the scree slopes of Rocky Top and Big Run Portal rise from the greenery.

Great Views

The white noise of Big Run resonates below as you repeatedly switchback down the stony path. Reach a concrete trail signpost, turn left, walk a few feet, and come to a second trail signpost at 4.9 miles. ►5 Stay left at the second trail marker, joining the Big Run Portal Trail. Traverse dense forest on a foot-friendly former fire road, then rock-hop Big Run, with its small pools and noisy cascades, at 5.1 miles. Alder bushes flank the trout stream, while witch hazel and sycamore shade gravel bars. Dogwoods add springtime color to the gorge. Make a second crossing at 5.6 miles. This crossing, like all the others in this watershed, can be dry-footed at normal water levels but is challenging when the water is high. Look for large white pines along the run. The evergreens have long, blue-green needles and evenly spaced branches. The gray vertically

Stream

Swimming

Big Run *flows crystalline along a gravel bar.*

peeling trunks of shagbark hickories are also easy to spot.

Make two easy crossings of Big Run in succession, then reach a trail junction at 6.3 miles. ▶6 Veer left on the Rocky Mountain Run Trail. It moderately ascends an old roadbed along Rocky Mountain Run, flanked with white pine, into a more intimate valley than Big Run. The path curves easterly at 6.7 miles. Normally dry tributaries bisect the path. Make your first easy crossing of Rocky Mountain Run at 7.2 miles. Watch for a slide cascade and plunge pool on your right at 7.7 miles. ▶7

Cross Rocky Mountain Run twice at 7.8 miles, and soon leave the roadbed. Large white oaks and tulip trees stand proudly overhead. Step over a tributary of Rocky Mountain Run at 8.0 miles. Look left here as the main stream flows over a rock slab. The

Waterfall

Stream

trail steepens and enters young spindly forest in a series of switchbacks, making a gap and trail junction at 8.9 miles. ►8 Turn right on the Brown Mountain Trail, and retrace your steps 0.6 mile farther, back to Brown Mountain Overlook at 9.5 miles. ►9

🚶 MILESTONES

►1	0.0	Brown Mountain Overlook at milepost 76.9
►2	0.6	Rocky Mountain Run Trail leaves left
►3	1.5	Great views from quartz outcrop
►4	3.7	Vista across Bearwallow Hollow
►5	4.9	Left on Big Run Portal Trail
►6	6.3	Left on Rocky Mountain Run Trail
►7	7.7	Waterfall
►8	8.9	Right on Brown Mountain Trail
►9	9.5	Brown Mountain Overlook at milepost 76.9

Loft Mountain Loop

To Swift Run Gap

Patterson Ridge Trail

Loft Mountain

Frazier Discovery Trailhead

79
5

Frazier Discovery Trail

P

Loft Mountain Wayside

Frazier Discovery Trail

Skyline Drive

SHENANDOAH NATIONAL PARK

To Rockfish Gap

Loft Mountain Camp Store

Loft Mountain Campground

N

| 0 | 0.2 | 0.4 | 0.6 mile |

| 0 | 0.2 | 0.4 | 0.6 kilometer |

Loft Mountain Loop

This loop is ideal for a family hike or an afternoon stroll. Start at the Loft Mountain Wayside, and take the Frazier Discovery Trail to a massive rock outcrop with an extensive view, where Loft Mountain opens to the heavens above and the lands below. Beyond the vista, pick up the world's most famous footpath, the Appalachian Trail (AT), southward through a transitional forest to meet a paved path near the Loft Mountain Campground camp store. Gently descend back to Loft Mountain Wayside. The hike is accessible for almost everyone, though the first part does climb to the rock outcrop.

Best Time

This hike is best enjoyed during the summer months in the cool of the high forest. Also, that is when the Loft Mountain Wayside (camp store) and Loft Mountain Campground are open. However, the vistas from atop Loft Mountain may be hazy then. Spring and fall are better for views. Winter presents extensive views and isolation.

Finding the Trail

Loft Mountain Wayside is located at milepost 79.5, on the west side of Skyline Drive. It is 26.1 miles north of Rockfish Gap Entrance Station. The Frazier Discovery Trail leaves from the wayside near the entrance to Loft Mountain Campground.

TRAIL USE
Day Hiking,
Pets Prohibited
LENGTH
2.9 miles, 2–3 hours
VERTICAL FEET
±450'
DIFFICULTY
– 1 **2** 3 4 5 +
TRAIL TYPE
Loop
START & FINISH
N38° 15.771'
W78° 39.634'

FEATURES
Ridgeline
Autumn Colors
Wildflowers
Great Views
Geological Interest

FACILITIES
Restrooms
Campground and
camp store
Picnic tables
Water

Trail Description

Leave the Loft Mountain Wayside, ►1 and cross Skyline Drive. Begin ascending a paved path, which is as much gravel and moss as pavement. Shortly intersect the Frazier Discovery Trail, turning left. You can purchase an interpretive booklet, adding to your hike. The dirt path splits; stay left again, and head uphill on a rocky slope shaded **Wildflowers** �֎ with hardwoods. This trail was once known as the "Deadening Trail," for the settlers' practice of girdling trees to kill them so that they could farm the land beneath the standing dead trees. It doesn't have quite the same ring as does Frazier Discovery Trail, which is named for the family that owned much of the area land, as well as a family that lived just below where Loft Mountain Wayside stands today. At 0.4 mile, curve beneath a big rock overhang on a **Geological Interest** ✐ rocky tread. ►2 The upthrust rock provides shelter for storm-bound hikers.

Keep uphill amid woods to emerge onto a rock outcrop jutting into the sky at 0.6 mile. ►3 Enjoy this panoramic view from 3,300 feet atop Loft Mountain. The peaks of Shenandoah National Park poke their heads upward to the west. Below, the Shenandoah Valley occupies the lowlands. Massanutten Mountain parallels the Blue Ridge upon which you stand. The

Loft Mountain Loop Elevation Profile

Alleghenies of West Virginia rise in the farthest hazy reaches. Floyd Frazier, one of the last of the Fraziers to reside in what is now the park, called this outcrop Raven Rocks. Loft Mountain was previously known as Frazier Mountain and Lost Mountain. The outcrop is very large. Walk about, enjoying the varied vistas, but please be aware of sensitive vegetation on the outcrop as you explore.

Great Views

Leave the rocky viewpoint, and at 0.7 mile turn right, southbound, onto the AT, concurrent with the Frazier Discovery Trail. Soon, a side trail leading right opens to a second vista. ►4 Go ahead and clamber on the rocks and determine if this view is superior to the first. The outcrop is smaller, yet higher. Patterson Ridge and Big Run are to the west. Big Flat Mountain and Loft Mountain Campground are due south. From this vantage, I once saw a mother bear and two cubs strolling the leafless forest below. Ahead, stay on the AT as the Frazier Discovery Trail leaves right. Many spindly, narrow-trunked trees crowd the AT. Locust and cherry trees indicate recent reforestation of pastureland where Frazier once tended cattle.

Almost the entire mountain crest here was a meadow. The cows grazed amid million-dollar views! Look for larger oak trees with widespread limbs amid the younger trees. The limbs on these older trees that once enjoyed sunlight are now denied light with reforestation, and some limbs are dying and breaking off. These older trees provided shade for the cattle when it was meadow. Parts of the trail pass through low briar-infested areas open to the sky. Keep forward on the AT beyond an over-grown road that once led 0.5 mile to the camp store. A concrete signpost still marks the intersection. The AT footbed becomes grassy beneath scraggly forest.

Ridgeline

At 1.8 miles, turn right on a narrow trail leading 75 yards to the Loft Mountain camp store. ►5 This turn is marked with a concrete signpost. Pass

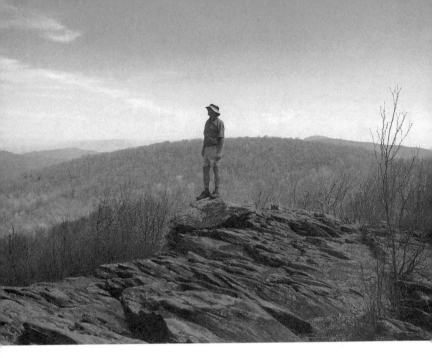

Loft Mountain *provides an early-spring panorama.*

behind the camp store; take advantage of its offerings if you are hungry or thirsty. Just past the store, turn right onto an unnamed paved trail. Gently descend on the crumbly path beneath hawthorn and locust trees that typically reclaim old fields. Look left of the trail for a water fountain made to appear as if the spigot is coming directly from the rock. Shortly pass the Frazier Discovery Trail a final time before reaching Loft Mountain Wayside at 2.9 miles, ending your loop. ▶6

🚶	MILESTONES	
▶1	0.0	Loft Mountain Wayside at milepost 79.5
▶2	0.4	Huge rock overhang
▶3	0.6	Great views from large outcrop atop Loft Mountain
▶4	0.7	Second vista, and join AT, southbound
▶5	1.8	Right at spur to camp store; pick up southbound paved track
▶6	2.9	Loft Mountain Wayside at milepost 79.5

Patterson Ridge Loop

This tough loop combines a remote wilderness trail, the park's biggest stream, some high country, and a campground. Start your hike on the seldom-trod Patterson Ridge Trail, rolling west along a ridge offering some views, then pass through a striking chestnut oak forest. Descend to Big Run, literally the biggest stream in the park. Turn up Big Run, rock-hopping your way along the watercourse, with its rich forest and rock walls, to reach the Big Run Loop Trail, which leads to Skyline Drive.

Cross the drive, and join the fabled Appalachian Trail (AT), heading northbound. Come near Loft Mountain Campground. End the hike by descending past the Loft Mountain camp store. The difficulty in this hike is based on the distance combined with elevation change, which amounts to a 1,500-foot drop, a 1,900-foot rise, and a final 400-foot descent back to the trailhead.

Best Time

This hike is best enjoyed from late spring through late fall. The crossings of Big Run are manageable then, and the trailhead facilities at Loft Mountain Wayside are open.

Finding the Trail

Loft Mountain Wayside is located at mile 79.5, on the west side of Skyline Drive. It is 26.1 miles north of Rockfish Gap Entrance Station. The Patterson Ridge Trail starts on the west side of Skyline Drive a little north of the Loft Mountain Wayside.

TRAIL USE
Day Hiking,
Backpacking
LENGTH
9.7 miles, 5.5–7 hours
VERTICAL FEET
±1,900'
DIFFICULTY
− 1 2 3 4 **5** +
TRAIL TYPE
Loop
START & FINISH
N38° 15.771'
W78° 39.634'

FEATURES
Ridgeline
Stream
Autumn Colors
Wildflowers
Great Views
Swimming
Secluded

FACILITIES
Campground and
camp store
Picnic tables
Restrooms
Water

Patterson Ridge Loop

Big Run

Rocky Mountain Run

Rocky Mountain Run Trail

To Swift Run Gap

Rockytop Overlook

Big Run Portal Trail

Patterson Ridge Trail

Skyline Drive

SHENANDOAH NATIONAL PARK

Big Run

79
.5

Loft Mountain Wayside

Big Run Loop Trail

Big Run Loop Trail

Big Run Overlook

Loft Mountain Camp Store

Loft Mountain Campground

Skyline Drive

Doyles River Overlook

To Rockfish Gap

Doyles River Trail

N

0   0.2   0.4   0.6 mile

0   0.2   0.4   0.6 kilometer

Trail Description

Start the hike by leaving Loft Mountain Wayside
▶1 and walking northbound along Skyline Drive
for approximately 50 yards. Pass the sign indicating
Loft Mountain Wayside for oncoming motorists,
then look left for the concrete post indicating the
Patterson Ridge Trail. Turn left here (a fire road
is across from you), and begin ascending a grassy
track, to soon level out in hickory–oak woods.
The westerly walking is easy on the well-groomed
yet lightly used path. Begin a steady but gradual
descent, making the first of many switchbacks at 0.6
mile. Occasional views break in partially canopied
areas, rife with sumac and locust.

 Ridgeline

At 1.0 mile, a view opens on a switchback.
▶2 Here, you can gander northwest through the
Big Run Portal to Massanutten Mountain, the
Shenandoah Valley, and the rock outcrops and
talus slopes of the lower Big Run Valley. The well-
groomed singletrack trail hastens downward only to
meet a gap at 1.1 miles and then climb. The ascent
eases as the Patterson Ridge Trail slips over to the
northeast side of the ridge. Obscured views of Rocky
Mountain and Rocky Mountain Run open. The path
levels out for some distance in gnarled oaks and
wind-sculpted pines before making a last climb to
a knob. Here, at 1.9 miles, the trail curves north
onto the dividing ridge between Big Run and Rocky
Mountain Run. Keep descending on the nose of
this ridge, passing through a striking forest of gray-
trunked chestnut oaks.

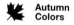 **Great Views**

The downhill accelerates. Be glad you aren't
going up this. The woods thicken after passing
through a wooded talus slope. Reach the Big Run
Portal Trail and the low point of the hike at 3.2
miles. ▶3 Turn left here, heading up the Big Run
Portal Trail. Big Run flows off to your right. Trace
an old fire road through plush woods where white
pines and white oaks prevail. The ascent is negligible

Autumn Colors

 Stream

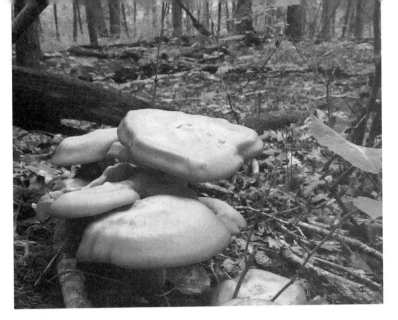

Wonders at Shenandoah *come in packages big and small, such as these woodland mushrooms.*

Wildflowers

Swimming

as you hike the wide valley. Intermittent wet weather tributaries cross the path. Watch for rock outcrops bordering Big Run. Rock-hop Big Run at 3.8 miles, as a rock bluff forces the trail to the right bank. Cross the stream again at 4.1 miles, just below a big pool where trout can be seen. A third crossing at 4.3 miles takes you back to the right bank, still ascending in woods dominated by tall white pines. The ascent picks up as you step over a tributary coming in from your right.

Patterson Ridge Loop Elevation Profile

At 4.7 miles, you curve south, up a tributary into a cove hardwood forest, where tulip trees rise regal and gray. Reach the Big Run Loop Trail at 5.2 miles. ▶4 Stay left here, as the Big Run Loop Trail passes an area where camping is prohibited and crosses the tributary you've been following. Watch for an overhanging rock shelter just beyond this crossing. Leave the sound of water behind while climbing into pine–oak–laurel woods on a slim mountainside path.

Crest out on a ridge dividing branches of Big Run at 5.6 miles. Gain views of the mountain crest on a short descent. Keep working for the high country, passing a streamlet. Crest out again at 6.7 miles, then make two wide, loping switchbacks, now aiming for Skyline Drive. Reach a signboard just before making the Big Run Overlook at 7.4 miles. ▶5 This overlook accessible by automobile presents palpable panoramas into Big Run. Keep north on Skyline Drive for 60 yards, reaching the Doyles Run Parking Area on the far side of the road.

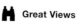 **Great Views**

Join the Doyles Run Trail and walk a few feet before meeting the AT. Turn left here, northbound on the AT, amid locust trees, cherry trees, and thick underbrush. Much of the area is open overhead. Keep a slight ascent. Look for occasional large oak trees with widespread limbs, indicating the former openness of the regenerating forest. Level out at 7.9 miles, and reach an outcrop with north and west views to Brown Mountain and Big Run watershed. ▶6 The path gently climbs, surmounting the 3,000-foot mark.

 Ridgeline

 Great Views

Meet a spur trail leading to the Loft Mountain camp store at 8.4 miles. ▶7 Stay left with the spur, as the AT leaves right, circling Big Flat Mountain. An uptick leads to a high point and the Loft Mountain Campground amphitheater at 8.6 miles. ▶8 You are entering the greater Loft Mountain developed area.

From the amphitheater, stay left downhill on a crumbly asphalt track to soon cross the Loft Mountain Campground road and reach the camp store at 8.8 miles. ▶9 Continue downhill on the asphalt path, paralleling the campground road. An easy decline leads you past the Frazier Discovery Trail to the Loft Mountain Wayside and the hike's end at 9.7 miles. ▶10

🚶 MILESTONES

▶1	0.0	Loft Mountain Wayside at milepost 79.5
▶2	1.0	View
▶3	3.2	Left on Big Run Portal Trail
▶4	5.2	Left on Big Run Loop Trail
▶5	7.4	Big Run Overlook
▶6	7.9	View
▶7	8.4	Left on paved spur toward camp store
▶8	8.6	Loft Mountain Campground amphitheater
▶9	8.8	Camp store
▶10	9.7	Loft Mountain Wayside at milepost 79.5

Big Run Loop

This circuit takes you through several types of forest and mountain lands. Start at Big Run Overlook, then descend into prototype oak woods. Travel a dry piney ridgeline with its attendant mountain laurel. Make your way to a tributary of Big Run, where a moist valley harbors cove hardwoods such as tulip trees. After climbing out, join a ridgeline that leads to the Appalachian Trail (AT), where you walk the spine of the Blue Ridge amid boulder fields and bluffs.

Best Time

This loop is good for spring wildflowers as it dips into the Big Run watershed. It is especially good for autumn colors since the circuit explores several forest types as it heads low and yet remains mostly level once it gets to the high country.

Finding the Trail

This hike leaves from the Big Run Overlook, on the west side of Skyline Drive at milepost 81.2. The Big Run Trail begins on the south side of the overlook.

Trail Description

Leave Big Run Overlook, ▶1 enthralling yourself with an unobstructed view of Shenandoah's biggest watershed while joining the Big Run Loop Trail. Descend the west slope of Blue Ridge on a slender singletrack path. The blue-blazed trail snakes beneath sturdy oaks, striped maple, hickory, witch hazel, and mountain laurel. Impressive boulders

TRAIL USE
Day Hiking

LENGTH
5.8 miles, 3.5–4.5 hours

VERTICAL FEET
±1,160'

DIFFICULTY
– 1 2 **3** 4 5 +

TRAIL TYPE
Loop

START & FINISH
N38° 15.224'
W78° 41.055'

FEATURES
Ridgeline
Stream
Autumn Colors
Wildflowers
Great Views
Historical Interest
Geological Interest

FACILITIES
None

 Great Views

Big Run Loop

SHENANDOAH
NATIONAL
PARK

Big Run Overlook

To
Swift Run
Gap

Skyline Drive

Doyles River Trail

Doyles River Overlook

Skyline Drive

Browns Gap Fire Road

Big Run Loop Trail

Big Run Portal Trail

Big Run Loop Trail

Big Run Loop Trail

Rockytop Trail

Madison Run Spur

Madison Run Fire Road

To Rockfish Gap

Browns Gap

N

0   0.1   0.2   0.3 mile
0   0.1   0.2   0.3 kilometer

are strewn about the rocky woods. At 0.2 mile, the path switchbacks right, dropping steadily. The trail briefly picks up a ridgeline before curving sharply left in a gap at 0.7 mile. Skirt around a watershed, crossing a wet-weather stream at 1.2 miles. Look for a small cascade on the lower end of the crossing. Oaks, hickory, and white pine dominate the woods, along with birch, representing both moist and dry forest flora. It seems a somewhat confused forest, a mix of species. However, the variety is really indicative of the incredible biodiversity of the Appalachians, rich in ecosystems that do not delineate perfectly from one another, but rather mix and meld forest habitats. The technical term is an overlapping of ecotones.

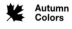
Autumn Colors

Soon, come to a second ridgeline. This crest is cloaked in pines, coloring the pathway gold with their needles. At 1.6 miles, traverse a gap and briefly climb. Quickly, you are descending. Watery sounds sing below. Come to a perennial tributary of Big Run at 2.2 miles. ▶2 Look for the overhanging rock shelter that could come in handy during a thunderstorm on your left before reaching the stream. Rock-hop the clear and cool watercourse. Take note that it divides into tributaries just above this crossing. Tulip trees, black birch, sugar maple, and other components of the cove hardwood forest predominate in this moist vale. You might want to

Stream

Wildflowers

Big Run Loop Elevation Profile

Tulip trees *rise in a cove hardwood forest.*

take a break here since this is the low point of the hike and you have a substantial climb ahead. This is also your only guaranteed opportunity to get water. There once was a trail shelter in the vicinity before the area became part of the Shenandoah Wilderness and the shelter was removed.

Meet a trail junction at 2.3 miles. ▶3 To your right, the Big Run Portal Trail leaves right for the lower valley of Big Run. Stay left on the Big Run Loop Trail, now cruising through a fern-floored forest of tulip trees. Oaks gain domain as you rise. Come along a wet-weather tributary you have been paralleling at 3.0 miles, just before turning sharply right. Continue a moderate uptick, rolling into a four-way trail junction at 3.5 miles. ▶4 The grassy gap begs a rest. That was a nearly 900-foot climb the last 1.3 miles! From here on the hike is relatively easy, with only moderate elevation changes.

Take a left at the intersection, still on the Big Run Loop Trail. This grass-lined track travels easterly and gently toward the crest of the Blue Ridge, shaded by ridgetop hickories and oaks. Pass through a section of young spindly woods rising from the fallen trunks of moth-damaged trees from decades past. Your final descent bisects former pastureland, now growing up in locust. The forest ecotones keep evolving.

Ridgeline ▲

Meet the AT at 4.2 miles. ▶5 Turn left here, northbound, in brushy forest full of vines, fire cherry, and tulip trees. Slice through a gateway of boulders before emerging onto and crossing Skyline Drive at 4.5 miles. The trail swings over the east side of the Blue Ridge, saddling alongside some impressive gray stone bluffs. Note the rockwork on the downslope side of the AT, keeping the pathway level. At 4.8 miles, the AT emerges onto the Doyles River Overlook. ▶6 This Skyline Drive vista presents easterly looks into the Doyles River watershed, bordered by Little Flat Mountain and Cedar Mountain. The view was used by Confederate soldiers, who placed guns here to cover their brethren camped at nearby Browns Gap.

The trail reenters woods on the north side of the overlook. The walking remains easy on the east slope below Skyline Drive. You pass north of the Big Run Overlook and your car, but the AT keeps north to a trail junction at 5.7 miles. ▶7 Here, turn left and walk a few feet to reach the Doyles River Parking Area just off Skyline Drive. From this parking area, walk south a short distance along Skyline Drive to the Big Run Overlook, completing the hike. ▶8

Geological Interest

Great Views

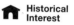
Historical Interest

🚶 MILESTONES

▶1	0.0	Big Run Overlook at milepost 81.2
▶2	2.2	Cross tributary of Big Run
▶3	2.3	Big Run Portal Trail leaves right
▶4	3.5	Stay left with Big Run Loop Trail at four-way junction and left again at next intersection
▶5	4.2	Left on the AT
▶6	4.8	Doyles River Overlook
▶7	5.7	Left to Doyles River Parking Area
▶8	5.8	Big Run Overlook at milepost 81.2

Rockytop and Big Run Loop

no public access
beyond this point

Brown
Mountain

Brown Mountain Trail

Rocky
Mountain

Lower Lewis Run

Big Run

Lewis Peak

Rocky Mountain Run

Lewis Peak Trail

Rockytop

Rocky Mountain Run Trail

Upper Lewis Run

Rockytop Trail

SHENANDOAH
NATIONAL
PARK

Big Run Portal Trail

Patterson Ridge Trail

Lewis Mountain Trail

Deep Run

Big Run

Austin Mountain Trail

Big Run Loop Trail

Rockytop Trail

To
Swift Run
Gap

Madison Run Fire Road

Skyline Drive

Doyles River

Madison Run

Browns Gap
Fire Road

N

To
Rockfish
Gap

83
.0

Browns
Gap

0   0.5   1   1.5 miles

0   0.5   1   1.5 kilometers

Rockytop and Big Run Loop

This loop takes you along the high ridge of Rockytop Mountain, where talus slopes and open boulders make for solitude-filled lookouts of the adjacent mountainscape and Shenandoah Valley beyond. Drop into crystalline Big Run, exploring the gorgeous valley of the park's largest watershed from low to high. The Big Run watershed is one of Shenandoah's finer backpacking destinations, even on the adjacent high ridges, where you must bring your own water.

Best Time

Since Big Run—the largest watershed in the park—has to be crossed numerous times, this circuit is best completed from late spring through late fall. Views are farthest reaching in spring and fall, but summer is best for fishing and swimming and enjoying the clear pools of Big Run.

Finding the Trail

The hike starts at the Browns Gap Parking Area at milepost 83.0 on Skyline Drive. From the Rockfish Gap Entrance Station, take Skyline Drive north for 21.6 miles to the trailhead, on your left.

Trail Description

Leave the Browns Gap Parking Area, ►1 and easily descend on Madison Run Fire Road. The Browns Gap Turnpike, built in 1805, originally laid out the modern gravel track you follow. Civil War

TRAIL USE
Day Hiking,
Backpacking
LENGTH
13.3 miles, 8–10 hours
VERTICAL FEET
±1,570'
DIFFICULTY
– 1 2 3 4 **5** +
TRAIL TYPE
Loop
START & FINISH
N38° 14.428'
W78° 42.654'

FEATURES
Ridgeline
Stream
Autumn Colors
Great Views
Swimming
Secluded
Steep
Historical Interest

FACILITIES
None

Excellent vistas *of the Shenandoah Valley open from the Rockytop Trail.*

Historical
Interest

Ridgeline ▲

troops crossed the Blue Ridge on the road in their Shenandoah Valley skirmishes. At 0.7 mile, after a sharp right turn, look for a trail marker on your right. ▶2 This is the Madison Run Spur Trail. Turn right and trace the spur uphill through pines 0.3 mile to a gap and a four-way trail junction. Turn left onto the Rockytop Trail. ▶3

Rockytop and Big Run Loop Elevation Profile

The path undulates along an oak–hickory ridge-top to arrive at yet another trail junction at 1.4 miles. ►4 Bear right, staying on the Rockytop Trail, as it slips around the east side of a knob while the Austin Mountain Trail stays left. The trail maintains a nearly level course, presenting views of the Blue Ridge and Big Run. Come to a sag at 2.0 miles, then swing to the southwest of another knob. The vegetation morphs to pine-mountain and laurel–oak woodland.

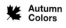
Autumn Colors

Bisect a rock field, and come to another gap. The trail then straddles the ridge while passing over a couple of small knobs. In summer, wildflowers color the understory. Views open to your east of Skyline Drive just before you meet the little-used Lewis Peak Trail at 3.3 miles. ►5 It is 1.1 miles to a worth-the-side-trip vista from Lewis Peak. Near here, wildland fires burned 1,150 acres in spring 2006. The trailside brush may still be overgrown.

This loop stays right with the Rockytop Trail. Begin descending seldom-trod track on loose stone. Confront an open sun-splashed scree slope at 3.6 miles. Nearby, a knob of Rockytop rises. This unnamed knob is actually higher than the Rockytop marked on topographic maps, which is where you are at this point. Beyond that, the Shenandoah Valley stretches across the flats. The southern tip of Massanutten Mountain rises as a backdrop. Drop from the scree into a gap at 4.0 miles. Curve around the slope of what many hikers refer to as the real Rockytop. Look back on the scree slope where you were, Lewis Peak to the southwest and Skyline Drive beyond. This Rockytop arguably offers better views than the first scree slope.

Secluded

Great Views

Enter a mix of rock and trees, the deposition of which allows more views to the west and north-west. Open onto breathtaking vistas of Shenandoah Valley at 4.7 miles while climbing away in switch-backs. Note the bigtooth aspen trees here atop the mountain. Drift through young woods and bands of

Steep 🧗

scree into a gap at 5.0 miles. Blueberries grow thick amid the rock, shrubby oaks, and squat pines. At 5.3 miles, the sandy trail drops in earnest toward Big Run. Until the low-slung sporadic forest grows back fully, enjoy nearly continuous views of the Shenandoah Valley below, pinpointing field, forest, and farm. Occasional switchbacks ease the single-track's downgrade.

Great Views 🔭

At 6.5 miles, reach a gap. ▶6 It is only 0.2 mile to the park boundary (where there is not public access). You turn right onto the Big Run Portal Trail, overlain on an old roadbed. The easy hiking is a relief after miles of loose stones and narrow tread. Descend in hickory–oak–laurel woods to span Big Run on a wide metal bridge at 7.0 miles. Enjoy looking at the stone slabs, pools, and gravel bars of the stream.

Stream 🌀

Pass the Brown Mountain Trail just beyond the bridge as you hike upstream in thick woods of maple, dogwood, witch hazel, and white pine aplenty. Alder bushes, green grasses, and splotchy sycamores rise along the watercourse. Rock-hop Big Run at 7.3 miles. Look up and downstream at canyon walls rising above the forest. In times of high flow, these crossings are challenging; use good sense. In summer, you will likely see more rock than water, allowing dry-shod crossings at normal water levels.

Autumn Colors 🍁

Big Run often braids around islands. Ahead, the trail follows a stony stream braid. Cross Big Run once again at 7.7 miles. The wide flats of this vale were once cultivated. Look for evidence of old-home sites, including walnut trees overtaking former fields. Cross Big Run at 8.2 and 8.3 miles in succession to reach a trail junction at 8.5 miles. ▶7 Big Run and Rocky Mountain Run come together here, forming a large and relatively flat drainage basin. Continue on the Big Run Portal Trail, rock-hopping Rocky Mountain Run and walking a peninsula between Rocky Mountain Run and Big Run. The

Swimming 🏊

Historical Interest 🏠

trail gradient remains mild. Intersect the Patterson Ridge Trail at 8.7 miles. ▶8 Stay on the Big Run Portal Trail under a green tunnel, crossing Big Run and its feeder streams several times.

At 10.3 miles, Big Run leaves left and the trail stays right, tracing a tributary under black birches. Meet the Big Run Loop Trail at 10.9 miles, in a lush cove of tulip trees. ▶9 You have gained 500 feet in the last 4.0 miles but now are fixing to ascend 1,100 feet in 2.0 miles. Take the fork to the right, climbing the steep trail along a slope, paralleling a tributary of Big Run. The Big Run Loop Trail switchbacks right at 11.6 miles, nearing the tributary before curving away into oak and mountain laurel woods. Reach a gap and familiar trail junction at 12.1 miles. ▶10 Turn left, staying on the Big Run Loop Trail as it ascends gently on a grass-lined track. Cross a brushy knob before intersecting the Appalachian Trail (AT) at 12.8 miles. ▶11 Turn right on the AT, and swing southward on an easy track. A mild downgrade in maples and oaks brings you to Browns Gap and the loop's end at 13.3 miles. ▶12

 Steep

♁	**MILESTONES**
▶1	0.0	Browns Gap Parking Area at milepost 83.0
▶2	0.7	Right on Madison Run Spur Trail
▶3	1.0	Left on Rockytop Trail
▶4	1.4	Right to stay on Rockytop Trail
▶5	3.3	Right to stay on Rockytop Trail as Lewis Peak Trail leaves left
▶6	6.5	Right on Big Run Portal Trail
▶7	8.5	Rocky Mountain Run Trail leaves left
▶8	8.7	Patterson Ridge Trail leaves left
▶9	10.9	Right on Big Run Loop Trail
▶10	12.1	Stay left on Big Run Loop Trail at gap
▶11	12.8	Right, southbound, on the AT
▶12	13.3	Browns Gap Parking Area at milepost 83.0

Austin Mountain and Madison Run Loop

Big Run Loop Trail

Big Run

To Swift Run Gap

Browns Gap Fire Road

Browns Gap

Big Run Loop Trail

Rockytop Trail

Madison Run Fire Road

Madison Run Spur Trail

Skyline Drive

Rockytop Trail

Dundo Overlook

Lewis Mountain Trail

Deep Run

Austin Mountain Trail

To Rockfish Gap

Madison Run

SHENANDOAH NATIONAL PARK

Austin Mountain

Whitcook Run

Madison Run Fire Road

0   0.2   0.4   0.6 mile

0   0.2   0.4   0.6 kilometer

N

Austin Mountain and Madison Run Loop

This lesser-hiked loop has plenty of rewards. Start at historic Browns Gap, tracing a modernized toll path, then join Austin Mountain Trail. This ridge-running trek takes you past clearings and over several talus slopes that avail seldom-seen outstanding views. Descend in pines to reach the valley of Madison Run, where rich forest shades a trout stream. Rejoin the roadbed and take it up the valley, winding along ridges and hollows back to Browns Gap.

TRAIL USE
Day Hiking,
Backpacking
LENGTH
8.8 miles, 5–6.5 hours
VERTICAL FEET
±1,260'
DIFFICULTY
− 1 2 3 **4** 5 +
TRAIL TYPE
Loop
START & FINISH
N38° 14.428'
W78° 42.654'

FEATURES
Ridgeline
Stream
Autumn Colors
Wildflowers
Great Views
Historical Interest

FACILITIES
None

Best Time

Every season has something to offer on this hike. Elevations are generally low, and the hike has no fords, making it a good winter option. In summer and fall, wildflowers proliferate along Madison Run Fire Road. Enjoy views on clear days during spring and autumn.

Finding the Trail

The hike starts at the Browns Gap Parking Area at milepost 83.0 on Skyline Drive. From the Rockfish Gap Entrance Station, take Skyline Drive north for 21.6 miles to the trailhead, on your left.

Trail Description

Leave Browns Gap beyond a chain gate, ▶1 descending gently on the Madison Run Fire Road. Many people have passed this way using what was Browns Gap Turnpike, built in 1805. Civil War troops crossed the Blue Ridge here. Since the edges of this

**Historical
Interest**

269

Wildflowers fire road are kept open, colorful summer and fall wildflowers, such as asters, line the way. The walking is easy on the smooth gravel track, unlike many other trails at Shenandoah National Park, and makes a good alternative for the foot-weary walker. Pines and oaks rise in the bordering woodlands, only partially shading the track. Madison Run is dropping sharply to your left. The road is used for fire management in this piney parcel of Shenandoah. Rangers also drive the track on patrol and access the western park lowlands.

At 0.7 mile, on a sharp right turn, look for a concrete signpost on your right that marks the Madison Run Spur Trail. ▶2 Leave the gravel track for a needle-carpeted foot trail, heading uphill. The fire road will be your return route. Follow the spur 0.3 mile to a gap and a four-way trail junction. Turn left on the ridge-running Rockytop Trail. ▶3 The grass-lined path ambles west among hickory, maple,

Autumn Colors oak, locust, and pin cherry.

Reach another trail junction at 1.4 miles. ▶4 Bear left on the Austin Mountain Trail, making a westward track far below an unnamed knob. The south-facing slope is cloaked in pines, azaleas, and

Ridgeline blueberries. Seclusion is yours. Usage drops off after each intersection, yet the path is well maintained, an advantage of being in Shenandoah National Park.

Austin Mountain and Madison Run Loop Elevation Profile

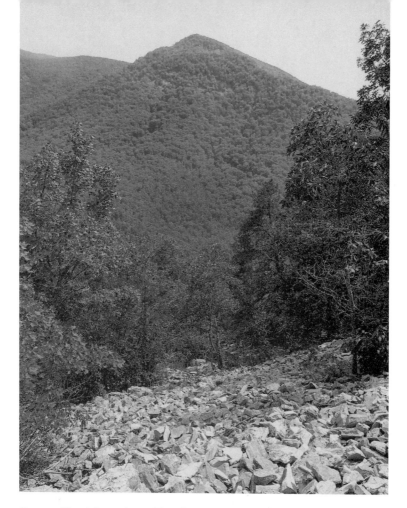

Furnace Mountain *stands proud from this Austin Mountain talus slope.*

The trailbed seems quite rocky after the smooth fire road. At 1.9 miles, in blueberries, look left for views of talus-sided Blackrock, a visible rock summit, wooded Trayfoot Mountain, and Furnace Mountain.

 Great Views

At 2.2 miles, the trail drops sharply down the spine of a ridge and then continues through grassy woodland. Make a sharp switchback to the left, and hit a gap at 2.6 miles. Work your way along the south side of Austin Mountain on an uptick. Absorb views of the Shenandoah Valley, then gaze back at

Great Views Dundo Overlook on Skyline Drive at 3.1 miles. ▶5
Reach the first of a series of talus slopes at 3.5 miles.
The high knob of Furnace Mountain stands directly
across Madison Run, and the lowlands can be seen
through the portal of Madison Run. Ahead, large
rock outcrops also offer vista points.

At mile 4.0, make a sharp switchback to the
left. The trail drops more than 500 feet in the next
half mile. Cross more talus, mixed with sporadic
tree cover, and join a wet-weather draw. Look for a
leveled area that once housed a dismantled and forgotten structure. Cross the wet-weather draw, then
Stream intersect the Madison Run Fire Road at 4.5 miles. ▶6

Wildflowers The fire road goes both directions. On the far
side of the woods flows Madison Run, a crystalline
stream with pools harboring brook trout. To complete the loop, head left on the fire road, wandering
up the wide, wooded flat. The road rises well above
the stream, allowing good looks of the water, especially when the valley tightens on this side of the
creek. At 5.2 miles, the track bridges a tributary
coming in from the left. A shaded grassy area lies
beside the stream. Follow the tributary vale where
tulip trees rise pencil straight toward the sky, along
with white oaks and red maple.

Continue climbing and make a big switchback
to the right. Begin a pattern of angling up midslope,
turning into tributaries of Madison Run that will
Autumn likely be dry, and then curving around dry ridges
Colors dividing them. These culverted tributaries come at
5.9, 6.2, 6.6, 7.0, and 7.3 miles. Beyond here, the
trail circles around a ridge and levels off at 7.5 miles,
even going down for a bit. ▶7 Grab some air because
the trail rises again. Complete the loop portion of
the hike at 8.1 miles. ▶8 You now have but 0.7 mile
and 150 feet of climbing ahead. Return to Browns
Gap at 8.8 miles, finishing the circuit. ▶9

🚶	MILESTONES	
▶1	0.0	Browns Gap Parking Area at milepost 83.0
▶2	0.7	Right on Madison Run Spur Trail
▶3	1.0	Left on Rockytop Trail
▶4	1.4	Left on Austin Mountain Trail
▶5	3.1	Begin series of great views
▶6	4.5	Left on Madison Run Fire Road
▶7	7.5	Level off on ridge
▶8	8.1	Complete loop and backtrack
▶9	8.8	Browns Gap Parking Area at milepost 83.0

Falls Loop from Browns Gap

Falls Loop from Browns Gap

Water lovers will fall for this loop. The trail passes three major cataracts and numerous other cascades as it explores two boulder-strewn canyons connected by the Appalachian Trail (AT). The hike up Jones Run passes some old-growth tulip trees with impressive girths. The trail grades are generally moderate. Add a little human history, and you have a great loop hike.

Best Time

This waterfall extravaganza is best in spring. The wildflowers offer up a colorful frame for the bold cataracts you will see. Summer is nice and cool but can be crowded, especially the Doyles River Trail. The streams will likely be low in autumn. Ice forms on the cascades during brisk winter days.

Finding the Trail

The hike starts at the Browns Gap Parking Area at milepost 83.0 on Skyline Drive. From the Rockfish Gap Entrance Station, take Skyline Drive north for 21.6 miles to the trailhead, on your left.

Trail Description

Cross Skyline Drive ▶1 and immediately begin descending on the Browns Gap Fire Road, the current name of the turnpike (Madison Run Fire Road, which leaves west from the gap near the parking area, is the western relic of this turnpike). Look for a small path leaving the road to your left at mile

TRAIL USE
Day Hiking,
Backpacking
LENGTH
7.0 miles, 4–5 hours
VERTICAL FEET
±1,280'
DIFFICULTY
– 1 2 3 **4** 5 +
TRAIL TYPE
Loop
START & FINISH
N38° 14.428'
W78° 42.654'

FEATURES
Ridgeline
Stream
Waterfalls
Autumn Colors
Wildflowers
Old-Growth Forest
Historical Interest
Geological Interest

FACILITIES
None

0.4. ▶2 Scramble a few feet up this path to the grave of William H. Howard, Confederate States of America soldier. The carved stone slab marks his grave. Return to the fire road, and continue down on a gentle grade, passing through a stand of pines. Views toward the Piedmont open through the trees.

Historical Interest

The wide track makes for easy walking. On your left at 0.9 mile, a brushy area contains relics indicating former human habitation such as piled rocks. ▶3 Imagine the forest as cleared and cultivated. As the trail swings to the left, the canopy of trees and oaks thickens. Watch for some large trailside trees, including a noteworthy tulip tree at 1.2 miles. Cross an iron bridge spanning sassy and shallow Doyles River. Reach a trail junction at 1.7 miles. ▶4

Stream

Turn right onto Doyles River Trail. Other hikers, who have come from Skyline Drive and the upper Doyles River Trailhead, will join you. The footpath descends along lively Doyles River. Cross the waterway, an easy rock-hop, at mile 1.9. This vale was once full of hemlocks, but an invasive insect known as the woolly adelgid killed them by sucking out their sap. The woolly adelgid is thought to have been introduced to the United States from Asia in 1924. Nearly all the hemlocks in the park have succumbed to this deadly pest, save for ones the park has treated with an insecticide injected into the ground below the trees.

Falls Loop from Browns Gap Elevation Profile

Hardwoods now dominate the forest. Wildflowers carpet the woodland floor.

Doyles River Trail continues along the watercourse but swings away as it approaches Upper Doyles Falls. At mile 2.1 a side trail leads to the dark pool at the base of the three-tier, 30-foot falls that drops into a bouldery glen at the point where a tributary feeds the river. ▶5 The canyon tightens; Doyles River makes frenzied drops. Unnamed cascades accompany you downstream until a sharp switchback leads to the base of Lower Doyles Falls at mile 2.4. ▶6 Lower Doyles Falls is the steeper and more spectacular of the two at 63 feet. It dives over a rock lip and then spills in ribbons, strands, and crashing channels over multiple tiers to finally land in a pool before charging on. The cataract looks different depending on the flow level. A rock wall extends across the far gorge.

Waterfall

The trail squeezes down the narrow, very rugged gorge, using a wooden bridge to span a cascading tributary spilling into Doyles River at 2.7 miles. At 2.9 miles, find a deep pool between quickly moving rapids. At 3.1 miles, in a small flat that would make a good lunch spot, come to a trail marker and the end of Doyles River Trail. ▶7 Jones Run and Doyles River merge below the signpost. Notice the sycamores in the lower valley—the climate is just too cold for them upstream on either branch.

Waterfall

Veer right on lesser-used Jones Run Trail, and begin to climb, rock-hopping Jones Run at 3.3 miles. ▶8 Impressive tulip trees grow tall with such wide diameters that it would take several hikers to encircle them. Look up the slope. Jones Run gorge is littered with huge boulders. Keep an eye on the creek too, as many scenic cascades tumble down the relentless watercourse, including some sliding cascades. At 3.8 miles, step over a tributary. ▶9 You arrive at Jones Run Falls, where water spills 45 feet over a solid rock wall. Large waterside rock slabs

Old-Growth Forest

Waterfall

Geological Interest

Ridgeline ▲

make for good observation points. Feel the cool air and mist from the cataract.

The trail turns sharply left, circumventing a rock rampart. Achieve the top of the falls. The path traces Jones Run past more cascades before veering away from the creek. Gently ascend through a cove hardwood forest with an open understory of grass and ferns. At 5.0 miles, join an old wagon road. The path widens. Step over Jones Run, minute at this point, at 5.2 miles. ▶10 Leave the wagon track, also heading for Browns Gap. The Jones Run Trail ascends and makes a sharp left turn at 5.4 miles.

Meet the AT at 5.7 miles. ▶11 The Jones Run Trailhead and Parking Area are just steps away. Turn right on the AT, northbound, toward Dundo Picnic Ground. Dry species, such as mountain laurel and chestnut oak, straddle the grade back to Browns Gap. Pass spur trails to Dundo Picnic Ground at 6.3 miles. ▶12 Intermittent views of Cedar Mountain open. The AT descends before arriving at Browns Gap. Complete your loop at 7.0 miles. ▶13

🚶 MILESTONES

▶1	0.0	Browns Gap Parking Area at milepost 83.0
▶2	0.4	Grave of Confederate soldier William H. Howard
▶3	0.9	Old-home site
▶4	1.7	Right on Doyles River Trail
▶5	2.1	Upper Doyles River Falls
▶6	2.4	Lower Doyles River Falls
▶7	3.1	Right on Jones Run Trail
▶8	3.3	Cross Jones Run
▶9	3.8	Jones Run Falls
▶10	5.2	Step over Jones Run
▶11	5.7	Right on the AT
▶12	6.3	Dundo Picnic Ground
▶13	7.0	Browns Gap Parking Area at milepost 83.0

Trayfoot Mountain Loop

Best Time

This long loop is excellent for backpacking but has a few fords, making it a late-spring–late-fall proposition. However, if doing it as a day hike, shoot for summer for maximum daylight.

Finding the Trail

From Rockfish Gap entrance station, drive north on Skyline Drive 20.5 miles to the Jones Run Parking Area, mile 84.1, on your right.

Trail Description

This long loop is best done as a two-night backpack. However, whether you execute this adventure as a very long day hike or a backpack, you will be well rewarded for your efforts. Combining the Appalachian Trail (AT), remote rock ridges, and mountain streams, this circuit hike presents views from multiple locations, allowing you to see where you are going and where you were. The hike's challenges will be felt in the two major climbs along its course. The first is the 2,000-foot rise from Madison Run up to Trayfoot Mountain, and the second is the 1,700-foot ascent from Paine Run to Blackrock, as well as lesser undulations along the ridges and the AT. Backpackers can divide the ups and downs, over-nighting at streamside campsites, whereas day hikers will be tested making the grades all in one day.

Start your loop northbound, departing the Jones Run parking area ▶1 on the AT. The hiking is easy as you pass beside Dundo Picnic Ground, which has

TRAIL USE
Day Hiking,
Backpacking
LENGTH
20.7 miles,
11–12.5 hours
VERTICAL FEET
±5,850
DIFFICULTY
– 1 2 3 4 **5** +
TRAIL TYPE
Loop
START & FINISH
N38° 13.791'
W78° 43.581'

FEATURES
Summit
Ridgeline
Stream
Autumn Colors
Wildlife
Great Views
Swimming
Secluded
Historical Interest
Geological Interest

FACILITIES
Picnic area along hike

Trayfoot Mountain Loop

This overlook *rewards hikers with vistas of Buzzard Rock and the Shenandoah Valley.*

water spigots and restrooms. Descend into Browns Gap at 1.3 miles, ▶**2** through which Stonewall Jackson traversed while he repeatedly bamboozled Yankees during the Civil War. Stay north with the AT, coming to a trail junction at 1.8 miles. Turn left on the Big Run Loop Trail, surmounting the Blue Ridge, then descend to another trail junction. Keep straight, joining the ridge-running Rockytop Trail, to bear left on the Austin Mountain Trail at 2.9 miles. ▶**3** The rocky track leads through pines, azaleas, and blueberries in solitude. At 3.4 miles, a view opens across Madison Run of the stony slopes of Blackrock Summit. Remember the spot; you will be there later. The wooded but stony Austin Mountain Trail opens to more views at 4.6 miles. Here you can peer west to the Shenandoah Valley, then gaze southeast to Dundo Overlook back on Skyline Drive. At 5.0 miles, the forest gives way to wide-open talus slopes, massive slopes of

 Historical Interest

 Ridgeline

 Secluded

You make two major climbs in one hike.

Geological Interest

Great Views

Stream

Swimming

Wildlife

Great Views

sun-burnished rock, revealing more panoramas. ▶4 Furnace Mountain rises across Madison Run. Ahead, additional rock outcrops present additional panoramas as you descend. At 5.5 miles, descend steeply after a sharp switchback. Step over a small streamlet before reaching Madison Run Fire Road at 6.1 miles. ▶5 Madison Run gurgles through the woods just beyond the fire road. Campsites and swimming holes can be found in the area. I have seen bears down here on numerous occasions. Hang your food if backpacking.

The loop turns right down Madison Fire Road, then left onto Furnace Mountain Trail at 6.7 miles. ▶6 Cross Madison Run on rocks, and continue downstream. Here begins your first big climb, working up Furnace Mountain, where breaks between scraggly pines, oaks, and outcrops deliver panoramas of the Shenandoah Valley. At 8.3 miles, you meet the side trail leading to the edge of Furnace Mountain. ▶7

Do not pass up this side trip. It leads 0.5 mile to a rock precipice on the side of Furnace Mountain. From this overlook, you can gaze across at where you were on Austin Mountain and below into the Madison Run watershed. Beyond the spur route, rejoin the pine- and mountain laurel–laced Furnace Mountain Trail. Pass through smaller scattered talus slopes before joining the Trayfoot Mountain Trail at 10.9 miles. ▶8

Trayfoot Mountain Loop Elevation Profile

Paine Run *can get low in summertime.*

The trail transforms from singletrack to double-track, reaching 3,374 feet atop Trayfoot Mountain Trail, at 11.1 miles. Beyond here, the path narrows again along the ridgecrest. You are going mostly downhill among oaks and other hardwoods. The farther you go, the more the path becomes rock and the more the forest transforms to primarily pine. Both aspects add scenic value, which you will see firsthand from a view at 13.4 miles. ▶9 Scope across Paine Run to Chimney Rock.

Continue the scenic downgrade, and reach a sharp left turn at 14.2 miles. Head to the outcrop at the turn, and walk out. Gander across Paine Run to Buzzard Rock, then outward to Shenandoah Valley beyond. Hike into Lefthand Hollow. A switchback takes you to Paine Run at 14.8 miles. ▶10 Reach the Paine Run Trail, and turn left, crossing the flat between Lefthand Hollow and Paine Run.

 Summit

▲ **Ridgeline**

 Great Views

Stream ▷◁

At 15.0 miles, hop over attractive and clear Paine Run on rocks. Hike through pine and mountain laurel forest on a moderate uptick. The trail repeatedly crosses feeder streams then returns to the main valley. Fragrant pines give way to rich hardwoods as you ascend the Paine Run Valley. The trail makes a sharp switchback to the right at 17.4 miles. ▶11 Here the old road to historic Blackrock Springs and a former resort site leads left. You might have to fight across a few fallen trees and through spider webs, but intrepid explorers will find building foundations, leveled spots, and springs where the resort operated for nearly a century.

The Paine Run Trail continues climbing, joining a xeric ridge to make Blackrock Gap at 18.3 miles. ▶12 Here, cross Skyline Drive, and head northbound on the AT to quickly cross Skyline Drive again. At 19.0 miles, meet the spur to stone Blackrock Hut and spring. ▶13

Great Views 🔭

Summit 🔺

The AT continues climbing as it circles Blackrock Summit. Incredible views open at 19.5 miles. ▶14 You can see where you have been—the vale of Paine Run, Austin Mountain, Furnace Mountain, Trayfoot Mountain, Madison Run, and the Shenandoah Valley beyond. (Please be mindful of sensitive vegetation on the outcrop as you explore.) This is the apex of the hike. From Blackrock Summit, keep north on the AT, passing the Blackrock Parking Area before crossing Skyline Drive a final time. Just a few minutes ahead is the Jones Run Parking Area, where you complete the rewarding trek at 20.7 miles. ▶15

🚶	**MILESTONES**	
▶1	0.0	Jones Run Parking Area
▶2	1.3	Browns Gap
▶3	2.9	Left on Austin Mountain Trail, views ahead
▶4	5.0	Talus slopes, views
▶5	6.1	Right on Madison Run Fire Road
▶6	6.7	Left on Furnace Mountain Trail
▶7	8.3	Spur to Furnace Mountain, vista
▶8	10.9	Right on Trayfoot Mountain Trail as Blackrock Trail leaves left, summit ahead
▶9	13.4	View, another view ahead in 0.8 mile
▶10	14.8	Left on Paine Run Trail
▶11	17.4	Spur to historic Blackrock Springs
▶12	18.3	Blackrock Gap, join AT
▶13	19.0	Spur to Blackrock Hut
▶14	19.5	Blackrock Summit, views
▶15	20.7	Jones Run Parking Area

SHENANDOAH
NATIONAL
PARK

Furnace
Mountain

Whiteoak Run

Madison Run Fire Road

Madison Run

Miller Run

Furnace Mountain Trail

To
Swift Run
Gap

84
.0
P
Jones Run
Parking Area

Snull Run

Trayfoot Mountain Trail

Trayfoot
Mountain

Trayfoot Mountain Trail

P
84
.8
Blackrock Summit
Parking Area

Blackrock
Summit

Skyline Drive

Pinestand
Mountain

N

0   0.2   0.4   0.6 mile
0   0.2   0.4   0.6 kilometer

To
Rockfish
Gap

Blackrock
Gap

Moormans River
Fire Road

Trayfoot Mountain
Overlook

Furnace Mountain via Blackrock

This outstanding hike shows off special features of Shenandoah, namely its interesting geology that results in huge outcrops rising above the forest and open talus slopes where rocks by the thousands carpet the mountainsides. Once you finish soaking in the outstanding views of Blackrock Summit with other hikers, enter one of the park's more remote areas, availing maximum solitude. Be careful because the trail is rocky. Take your time and enjoy the solitude of Furnace Mountain.

Best Time

Take this view-laden trek when the skies are clear. You will be amply rewarded.

Finding the Trail

The Blackrock Parking Area is located at milepost 84.8 on Skyline Drive, on the west side. From the Rockfish Gap Entrance Station, it is a 19.9-mile drive to the trailhead.

Trail Description

Leave the Blackrock Parking Area, ▶1 passing around a pole gate on the wide roadbed of the Trayfoot Mountain Trail. Locust, ferns, and grasses border the track. Begin climbing and intersect the slender, shady Appalachian Trail (AT) at 0.1 mile. ▶2 Head left, south, on the level-running master path of Shenandoah. The Trayfoot Mountain Trail runs parallel to the AT at this point and is within

TRAIL USE
Day Hiking,
Backpacking
LENGTH
6.8 miles, 4–5 hours
VERTICAL FEET
±900'
DIFFICULTY
− 1 2 **3** 4 5 +
TRAIL TYPE
Out-and-back
START & FINISH
N38° 13.370'
W78° 44.010'

FEATURES
Summit
Ridgeline
Autumn Colors
Great Views
Secluded
Geological Interest

FACILITIES
None

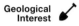
sight. It isn't long before the woods give way and you enter the open stones of Blackrock. ▶3 To your left, huge boulders rise in crazy formations, making for exciting scrambling opportunities. To your right, a gray talus slope recedes down the mountain, opening up stupendous highland panoramas. Furnace Mountain, your destination, rises to the west. Madison Run cuts a wooded swath between Austin Mountain and Furnace Mountain. The valley is known as Dundo Hollow. Austin Mountain forms a rampart to the north. More peaks rise in the distance, while the Shenandoah Valley fades to the horizon. This is one of the finest spots on the AT, in my opinion. (Please be aware of sensitive vegetation as you walk around.)

The AT curves left to intersect the Blackrock Spur Trail at 0.4 mile. ▶4 Turn right, joining the spur. Make a stony passage through boulders, opening onto a rocky ridge with plentiful panoramas, limited only by how many outcrops you want to visit. Trailside views are numerous too. Trayfoot Mountain stands brazen, with its talus slopes forming breaks in the forest. The valley of Paine Run falls away to your left. This is a place to linger. Trees eventually overtake the protuberance, and you intersect the Trayfoot Mountain Trail at 0.7 mile. ▶5

Turn right on the Trayfoot Mountain Trail, traveling westerly on a slender ridge. Enter the

Great Views

Furnace Mountain via Blackrock Elevation Profile

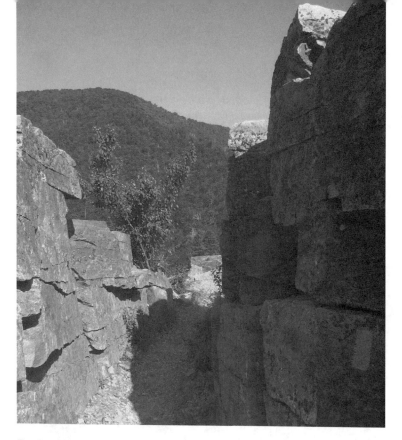

Trayfoot Mountain Trail *squeezes between stone ramparts en route to Furnace Mountain.*

Shenandoah Wilderness, though you will note no difference, save for lack of other hikers. Note the lesser-used trailbed. Reach a gap, then begin climbing a grassy ridge bordered with brushy, younger locust, sumac, and blackberries. This area was hit hard by the gypsy moth, which defoliated trees. They were introduced to the northeastern United States from Europe in 1869. The insects reached Shenandoah in 1983 and wrought havoc; their legacy still can be seen three decades later.

▲ **Ridgeline**

Ascend to an intersection at 1.3 miles. ▶6 Here, it is but 0.2 mile to the summit of Trayfoot Mountain. You are at the high point of this hike, above 3,000 feet. Leave the Trayfoot Mountain

Autumn Colors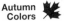

Trail, and turn right on the Furnace Mountain Trail. I have never seen another hiker past this point. Oak halls, along with hickories and low-slung sassafras, shade the path. Drop off the northern flank of Trayfoot Mountain, and pass through a talus slope. The loose rock makes for tough footing. The trail loses elevation steadily, making two sharp turns, first to the left, then to the right. Arrive at a gap at 2.3 miles. The ridge narrows here as you cross an

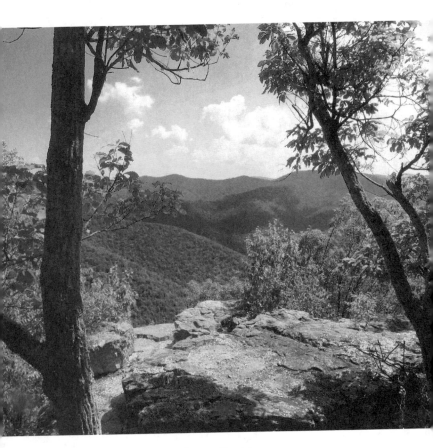

Looking north *from the outcrop at Furnace Mountain*

open forest of oaks, pines, and mountain laurel. Blueberries form a ground cover and ripen in July.

Surmount a knob, then meet the side trail to Furnace Mountain summit at 3.0 miles. ►7 Turn right on the spur trail, and begin climbing through pine–oak and laurel, mixed in with burnished quartz. As you ascend, wide views of the Shenandoah Valley open to your left. Bisect a small scree slope at 3.2 miles, then level off in a flat.

Descend slightly from the small wooded flat on the north side of Furnace Mountain to reach a distended rock outcrop. ►8 Here you can overlook the lower canyon of Madison Run in Dundo Hollow. Directly across the canyon stands Austin Mountain. Rockytop rises behind Austin Mountain. The main crest of the Blue Ridge stretches to your right. Relax and enjoy the view; you'll most likely have it all to yourself.

 Summit

 Great Views

🚶	**MILESTONES**	
►1	0.0	Blackrock Parking Area at milepost 84.8
►2	0.1	Left on the AT
►3	0.3	First-rate view from Blackrock
►4	0.4	Right on Blackrock Spur Trail
►5	0.7	Right on Trayfoot Mountain Trail
►6	1.3	Right on Furnace Mountain Trail
►7	3.0	Right on spur to Furnace Mountain summit
►8	3.4	Furnace Mountain summit

Blackrock Loop

SHENANDOAH
NATIONAL
PARK

Trayfoot Mountain Trail

Blackrock
Summit

Blackrock
Spur Trail

Blackrock Summit
Parking Area

84
.8

Skyline Drive

To Swift Run
Gap

To
Rockfish
Gap

Pinestand
Mountain

N

0   0.1   0.2   0.3 mile

0   0.1   0.2   0.3 kilometer

Blackrock Loop

Shenandoah is known for its overlooks and vistas. Many can be accessed from Skyline Drive. But, as hikers know, the best views are earned on foot. Not everyone can tramp for miles to an overlook. However, this short loop around the summit of Blackrock is doable by just about everyone from 4 to 84.

Start at nearly 3,000 feet, then make your way up the Trayfoot Mountain Trail on a wide track, topping a hill. Meet the Appalachian Trail (AT) and follow it northbound. Open onto an incredible rock jumble. Views extend for miles in multiple directions. Kids enjoy scrambling over massive boulders to reach the summit of Blackrock. Adults can stay on the AT. After gaining views from several spots, reenter woods, working your way back to the trailhead.

Best Time

This child-friendly highland walk is best whenever the skies are clear, whether it is winter, spring, or fall. Summer is often hazy, yet has its share of clear days. Also, the optional rock scrambling atop Blackrock is safest when the terrain is dry.

Finding the Trail

The Blackrock Parking Area is located at milepost 84.8 on Skyline Drive, on the west side of the road. From the Rockfish Gap Entrance Station, it is a 19.9-mile drive to the trailhead.

TRAIL USE
Day Hiking,
Child-Friendly
LENGTH
1.1 miles, 1–1.5 hours
VERTICAL FEET
±165'
DIFFICULTY
– **1** 2 3 4 5 +
TRAIL TYPE
Loop
START & FINISH
N38° 13.370'
W78° 44.010'

FEATURES
Summit
Ridgeline
Autumn Colors
Great Views
Geological Interest

FACILITIES
None

Trail Description

A large sign at the hike's beginning ▶1 details the tightly woven trail network lacing the crest of Blackrock. You walk under a mixed canopy of locust and other hardwoods. The large flowering black cohosh exhibits its fragrant white cylindrical flowers in midsummer. To the left of the trail, brushy woods proliferate. Look for blackened trunks of trees from a past fire. Curve uphill then come to the AT at 0.1 mile. ▶2 A few short steps connect the AT to the Trayfoot Mountain Trail here. For now, stay straight on the wide Trayfoot Mountain Trail, resuming an uptick, topping out at 0.3 mile. A hill rises yet higher to your left. Observe how the trail was used as a fire line. To the left, you can see old blackened trunks amid the regrowth, whereas to the right of the trail the woods exhibit no signs of burn within the past decade.

The slope opens to your left. Juicy blackberries attract man and beast alike. At 0.5 mile, come to a four-way intersection. ▶3 Here you meet the AT yet again. Turn right, northbound, on the AT. Soon you open onto the south side of the rock jumble that is Blackrock.

Hundreds, perhaps thousands of broken stones rise in a pile prescribed by the hands of God. Views open to the south, then west. Paine Hollow creates a void below, while the forest and rock slopes of

Autumn Colors

Ridgeline ▲

Geological Interest

Blackrock Loop Elevation Profile

Trayfoot Mountain rise in the distance. The boulder stack of Blackrock rises to your right. The stones of Blackrock are grayish, but a dark lichen known as rock tripe grows on them, giving them a dark appearance from afar. It will be hard to keep active kids from scaling the boulders. Maybe you should join them. (Please be aware of the sensitive vegetation growing on the rocks, though.) The view spreads 270 degrees from the top!

 Great Views

 Summit

Intersect the Blackrock Spur Trail at 0.6 mile. ▶4 More interesting geological formations, including mammoth boulder "gates" through which you walk, are down that trail. This loop stays with the AT as it continues circling Blackrock. A more accessible rock outcrop—as opposed to the jumble above you—stretches left toward Trayfoot Mountain.

As you turn north, a talus slope falls hundreds of feet down the mountain, revealing a wealth of national park beyond. Furnace Mountain forms a knob to the west. The talus slope drops to Madison Run below. Austin Mountain constructs a wooded wall across Madison Run. More Shenandoah highlands meld into the horizon, while the Shenandoah Valley flanks the lowlands below. Pull up a boulder and soak in the vista.

 Great Views

Leave the open rock expanse for the shady, singletrack, fern-bordered AT. The walking is easy and level. It isn't long before you meet the short spur to the wide Trayfoot Mountain Trail and complete your loop. From there, backtrack to the parking lot, completing the walk. ▶5

🚶 MILESTONES

▶1	0.0	Blackrock Parking Area at milepost 84.8
▶2	0.1	Pass the AT
▶3	0.5	Right on the AT
▶4	0.6	Blackrock Spur Trail leaves left
▶5	1.1	Blackrock Parking Area at milepost 84.8

Big Branch Falls via Moormans River

To Swift Run Gap

Skyline Drive

Blackrock Gap

87 4

Trayfoot Mountain Overlook

Paine Run

Moormans River Fire Road

N. Fork Moormans River

private trail

Paine Run Trail

SHENANDOAH NATIONAL PARK

Horsehead Mountain Overlook

Tobacco House Hollow

Little Gale Branch

Shop Run

Skyline Drive

N. Fork Moormans River Trail

N. Fork Moormans River

Big Branch

Pasture Fence Mountain ▲

To Rockfish Gap

Big Branch Falls

N

0   0.2   0.4   0.3 mile

0   0.2   0.4   0.6 kilometer

Big Branch Falls via Moormans River

This waterfall is rarely accessed from Skyline Drive, so this trek is filled with solitude. Most visitors start from Charlottesville Reservoir, making their way up to Big Branch Falls. Start on Skyline Drive, and descend to the North Fork Moormans River. Cruise along the scenic stream with cascades and pools in a deep valley bordered by high ridges. Everywhere-you-look beauty overlays this gorge bordered by Pasture Fence Mountain on one side and the Blue Ridge on the other. Finally, climb along low-flowing Big Branch, with its open watery bowls divided by rock slabs where the stream flows in slide cascades.

Best Time

Big Branch Falls are their best when the water is up, but since you must cross North Fork Moormans River, you don't want the water too high. Therefore, midspring–midsummer is best.

Finding the Trail

The Moormans River Fire Road begins at Blackrock Gap at milepost 87.4 on Skyline Drive.

Trail Description

Your hike leaves Blackrock Gap, elevation 2,330 feet, ►1 to moderately descend on the Moormans River Fire Road. The Appalachian Trail (AT) is just to your right. At 0.1 mile, step over a small branch that the trail begins to parallel.

TRAIL USE
Day Hiking,
Backpacking

LENGTH
7.6 miles, 4–5 hours

VERTICAL FEET
±880'

DIFFICULTY
– 1 2 3 **4** 5 +

TRAIL TYPE
Out-and-back

START & FINISH
N38° 12.395'
W78° 44.973'

FEATURES
Stream
Waterfall
Autumn Colors
Wildflowers
Swimming
Secluded

FACILITIES
None

Pass through pine, black gum, oak, and hickory woodland with an understory of mountain laurel, descending gently on the wide doubletrack. The branch you crossed drops steeply for North Fork Moormans River.

Autumn Colors

At 1.1 miles, come to a gate on the road; you are leaving the park for a period. ▶2 The trail stays on a right-of-way, descending to a junction at 1.4 miles. Turn right and immediately cross the North Fork Moormans River on rocks. ▶3 At higher flows this crossing may be a ford. The trail follows the river downstream. Look for ironwood and black birch in this deep vale. Wildflowers color the trailside in spring. At 1.6 miles, when a private road splits left, you stay right, passing a ramshackle hunter's camp on your left. Look for the smooth gray trunks of the many beech trees that grow in the area. Their nuts are a favored wildlife food source.

Stream

Wildflowers

Make another rock-hop of the river at 2.0 miles. ▶4 You stay on the west bank for the remainder of the hike. Bisect a small grassy clearing. Reenter the park at the crossing of Little Gate Branch at 2.1 miles. ▶5 The road takes on a more overgrown appearance and is now called the North Fork Moormans River Trail. Tightly growing, spindly trees are rising from what once was barren soil, remnants of a cataclysmic

Big Branch Falls via Moormans River Elevation Profile

Morning light breaks *on the North Fork Moormans River en route to Big Branch Falls.*

flood back in the 1990s. I saw this valley then, and the reforestation is truly amazing.

Cross Shop Run at 2.3 miles. The metal remnants of an old bridge lie in state here. Before the 1995 flood, Shenandoah National Park maintained this trail as a fire road. Step over an unnamed perennial stream at 2.7 miles. Come back along North Fork Moormans River at 2.9 miles. Tulip trees and syca- mores rise from the streamside. Gigantic boulders, gravel bars, speedy shoals, and quiet pools—some deep enough for a dip—all intermingle below.

 Swimming

Streamside open rock slabs beckon a visit. Brook trout, rock bass, and smallmouth bass ply the waters.

Stream ⮒

Come to Big Branch at 3.7 miles. ▶6 You can see the lower drops of Big Branch Falls from the main trail. Step over the stream, then take the 0.1-mile side trail that leads right to the falls. This canyon was also gouged back in '95, exposing the rock bed of the creek, making the entire scene more dramatic. The low-volume cataract drops 30 feet into a plunge pool, then another cascade slides into a second pool. Still another drop, the lowermost, dips into the deepest pool. As you explore the falls, ▶7 avoid slick spots on the open rock slabs adjacent to the moving water.

Waterfall ◤◥

🚶 MILESTONES

▶1	0.0	Blackrock Gap Parking Area at milepost 87.4
▶2	1.1	Leave park at a gate
▶3	1.4	Turn right and cross North Fork Moormans River
▶4	2.0	Cross North Fork Moormans River again
▶5	2.1	Reenter park at Little Gate Branch
▶6	3.7	Cross Big Branch
▶7	3.8	Big Branch Falls

Moormans River Loop

Best Time

This long loop is best for backpacking. It does have several fords, so early summer–late fall is the favored period.

Finding the Trail

From Rockfish Gap entrance station, drive north on Skyline Drive 14.6 miles to the Riprap Parking Area, at milepost 90.0 on your left.

Trail Description

This long circuit on the park's south side leads atop the Blue Ridge on the incomparable Appalachian Trail (AT) before dropping into the upper Moormans River watershed, where you walk along both scenic forks of the Moormans River. The loop then returns to the Blue Ridge, where you once again join the AT back to the trailhead. Highlights include Shenandoah panoramas not far from the trailhead, the North Fork Moormans River valley and its big pools, and Big Branch Falls. The South Fork Moormans River reveals more cascades and serene pools that attract bathers in summer. No matter what time of year, you will be forced to cross the above streams numerous times, so low-water times of the year (summer and fall) are best. Trekking poles or a hiking stick can help. Furthermore, though most of the hike is remote and secluded, the area near the Charlottesville Reservoir—also known as Sugar Hollow Reservoir—can be busy during

TRAIL USE
Day Hiking,
Backpacking

LENGTH
18.3 miles, 10–12 hours

VERTICAL FEET
±4,030

DIFFICULTY
– 1 2 3 4 **5** +

TRAIL TYPE
Loop

START & FINISH
N38° 10.662'
W78° 45.907'

FEATURES
Ridgeline
Stream
Waterfall
Autumn Colors
Wildflowers
Wildlife
Great Views
Swimming
Secluded
Historical Interest

FACILITIES
None

Moormans River Loop

Horsehead
Mountain

Paine Run

Paine Run Trail

Blackrock
Gap

To
Swift Run
Gap

North Fork
Moormans
River

Chimney
Rock

Riprap Trail

Little Gate
Branch

Rocks
Mountain

Riprap Trail
Parking Area

90.0

Big Branch

Pasture
Fence
Mountain

Big Branch
Falls

SHENANDOAH
NATIONAL
PARK

North Fork Moormans River

North Fork Moormans River Fire Road

Wildcat Trail

Crimora
Lake

Skyline Drive

Alt

Charlottesville
Reservoir

614

N

Turk Gap Trail

South Fork Moormans River

South Fork Moormans River Fire Road

Turk
Mountain

Turk
Gap

Middle
Mountain

Turk Mountain Trail

Turk Branch Trail

chimney
foundation

To
Rockfish Gap

0   0.5   1.0   1.5 miles

0   0.5   1.0   1.5 kilometers

Ruins like these *add historical value to the hike.*

summer with nearby residents beating the heat by dunking in the river pools.

The loop starts at the Riprap Parking Area, ▶1 but you trace the Riprap Trail only a few feet to join the AT, northbound, winding through shortish oaks. At 0.4 mile, the Riprap Trail leaves left, but you stay with the AT, ▶2 rolling along the Blue Ridge. Ahead, views open of Pasture Fence Mountain to the east and the Moormans River far below. You will be down there later. At 1.1 miles, after a descent, cross

Swimming

Enjoy national park-level scenery, plus chances to get wet.

Moormans River Loop Elevation Profile

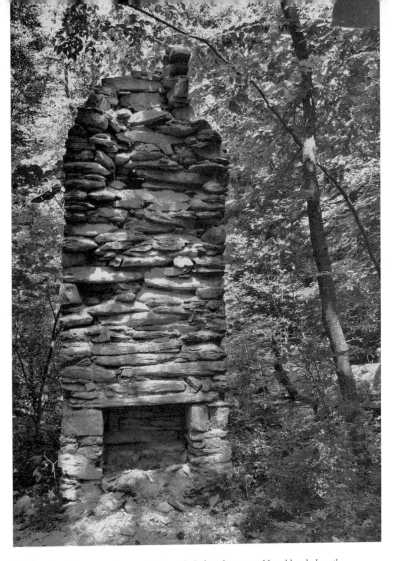

Pre-park settlers *spent many a chilly night before this now cold and lonely hearth.*

Ridgeline ▲

Skyline Drive. ▶3 Follow the AT as it circles around the east side of a knob to come near Skyline Drive in a gap. The trail stays on the east side of the scenic motor road. A few ups and downs on the ridgecrest give way to a descent in rocky woods. At 2.9 miles, reach Blackrock Gap. ▶4 The hike leaves the AT right, joining the gated and yellow-blazed North

Fork Moormans River Fire Road. The doubletrack makes for easy walking through national park–level scenery. Hop over a tributary of the Moormans River, then run parallel to the watercourse. At 4.0 miles, pass around a gate and temporarily leave the park. ▶5 At 4.3 miles, come to an intersection and the North Fork Moormans River. ▶6 Turn right to nimbly rock-hop the North Fork, your first of several crossings. Continue down the river valley on the main doubletrack. Stay right at a second junction after passing ramshackle hunt camps. At 4.8 miles, hop over the river again.

A gate and Little Gate Branch mark your reentry into Shenandoah National Park at 5.0 miles. ▶7 The track reverts to standard hiking trail. The next mile or so offers good backpack camps, along with alluring swimming holes made for a sultry Virginia summer afternoon. At 6.6 miles, step over Big Branch. ▶8 Below the crossing, a small waterfall tumbles toward North Fork Moormans River. However, a side trail leads right, upstream, 0.1 mile to the official Big Branch Falls. This 60-plus-foot spiller plunges over a series of naked rock slabs divided by clear pools. Check it out. Onward, the hike resumes tracing the North Fork Moormans River, flowing among massive boulders and beneath imposing bluffs. The trail is busier here, with hikers coming to Big Branch Falls from the parking area at Charlottesville Reservoir.

At 7.4 miles, rock-hop North Fork Moormans River. The path stays alongside the waterway. At 8.0 miles, dance across the river twice in succession, skirting a bluff. The North Fork Moormans River valley widens, and the trail soon leaves the national park, marked with vehicle barrier boulders. Keep straight on a gated road to reach VA 614 and a parking area at 8.8 miles. ▶9 This area can be confusing, so pay attention.

From the parking area, as VA 614 climbs left, you angle right on the gated South Fork Moormans

 Stream

 Swimming

 Waterfall

 Wildflowers

River Fire Road. Descend with the waterway to your right and shortly reach a concrete ford, crossing North Fork Moormans River a final time near the Charlottesville Reservoir, also known as Sugar Hollow Reservoir. The trail turns up along North Fork, away from the reservoir, then angles south, entering the South Fork Moormans River valley. Step over smaller South Fork at 9.7 miles. At 10.2 miles, in a wooded flat, come upon a pioneer homesite complete with a standing chimney. ▶10 As you push upstream, you'll come upon a huge rock outcrop to the left of the trail with a deep pool in the river below an angled cascade to your right. To top it off, a deeper pool and bigger waterfall are just ahead. It is hard not to stop and enjoy the South Fork Moormans River in these parts.

Beyond the pools you will find a stone home foundation and a long stone fence, site of another homesite. At 10.7 miles, hop what is left of South Fork Moormans River. Soon, fully reenter the park past a gate. At 10.9 miles, come to the Turk Branch Trail, ▶11 marked with the signature Shenandoah National Park concrete signpost. Additionally, a USGS survey marker has been embedded into a boulder at the intersection.

The loop leaves the South Fork Moormans River, heading right on the Turk Branch Trail. At 11.2 miles, pass an old-home site and step over Turk Branch. Look for road-leveling stonework from pre-park days. The path climbs alongside a tributary of Turk Branch, crossing it twice near more stonework. The trail then curves uphill, returning to cross now-small Turk Branch at 12.2 miles. ▶12 That's it for trailside water. Climb among mountain laurel and pines, coming near Skyline Drive. The pathway then parallels Skyline Drive before reaching the Turk Gap Parking Area at 13.4 miles. Cross the small paved lot, then meet the Appalachian Trail. Take the

Stream 🌊

Historical Interest 🏠

Swimming 🏊

Wildflowers 🌼

Secluded 👤

famed trail northbound under a canopy of oaks. ▶13
After your climb up Turk Branch, enjoy the mostly
level AT before descending to cross Skyline Drive at
15.3 miles. ▶14 The walking remains easy. At 15.6
miles, meet the Wildcat Trail. ▶15 Stay with the AT
under a low and often-open pine canopy.

▲ **Ridgeline**

This very dearth of trees in places allows westerly panoramas of the Shenandoah Valley before the
AT crosses over to the east side of the Blue Ridge.
Curve around the ridgeline to the right, and climb,
meeting the Riprap Trail at 18.3 miles. Turn right
and walk just a few feet to the Riprap Parking Area,
completing the circuit. ▶16

 Great Views

🚶	**MILESTONES**	
▶1	0.0	Leave Riprap Parking Area
▶2	0.4	Riprap Trail leaves left; stay with AT
▶3	1.1	Cross Skyline Drive
▶4	2.9	Blackrock Gap, right on North Fork Moormans River Fire Road
▶5	4.0	Pass around gate
▶6	4.3	Right at intersection, cross North Fork
▶7	5.0	Gate, reenter park
▶8	6.6	Big Branch Falls
▶9	8.8	VA 614 parking lot
▶10	10.2	Pass chimney
▶11	10.9	Right on Turk Branch Trail
▶12	12.2	Last trailside water
▶13	13.4	Turk Gap, right on AT
▶14	15.3	Cross Skyline Drive
▶15	15.6	Wildcat Trail leaves left; stay with AT
▶16	18.3	Return to trailhead, completing loop

Chimney Rock

Paine Run

Paine Run Trail

To Swift Run Gap

Skyline Drive

Horsehead Mountain Overlook

SHENANDOAH NATIONAL PARK

Chimney Rock

Calvary Rocks

Riprap Trail

Skyline Drive

Riprap Trail Parking Area

To Rockfish Gap

Big Branch

N

0   0.1   0.2   0.3 mile

0   0.1 0.2   0.3 kilometer

Chimney Rock

Be careful when you get to Chimney Rock. A deep crevasse separates the actual Chimney Rock and the rock you can reach safely. At one time a short bridge spanned this crevasse, but only the metal anchors remain. The bridge was removed when the Shenandoah Wilderness was created. This wilderness adds a layer of extra protection to large disjunct tracts of land within the park.

Since the bridge to the Chimney Rock was not part of the natural landscape, it was removed. However, the views are still stellar from the outcrop adjoining Chimney Rock, as well as a point along the route to Chimney Rock.

Best Time

This hike is a winner any time of year—the exposed quartz is interesting close-up. But the views from the outcrops are at their finest in spring, fall, and on clear winter days.

Finding the Trail

The Riprap Parking Area is located at milepost 90.0 on the west side of Skyline Drive, 14.6 miles north of the Rockfish Gap Entrance Station.

Trail Description

The hike starts on the Riprap Trail. Leave the Riprap Parking Area, ▶1 and walk a grand total of 83 feet before intersecting the Appalachian Trail (AT). Turn right on the AT, northbound, and climb north

TRAIL USE
Day Hiking,
Backpacking
LENGTH
3.4 miles, 2–3 hours
VERTICAL FEET
±480'
DIFFICULTY
– 1 **2** 3 4 5 +
TRAIL TYPE
Out-and-back
START & FINISH
N38° 10.665'
W78° 45.908'

FEATURES
Ridgeline
Autumn Colors
Great Views
Geological Interest

FACILITIES
None

The Shenandoah Valley *stretches west as far as the clarity of the sky allows.*

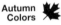

**Autumn
Colors**

through a pine–oak forest with a thick understory of azaleas, serviceberries, and mountain laurel. The evergreen mountain laurel shrubs display their pink blooms in May and June. The AT is in excellent shape here, despite the stony terrain.

Chimney Rock Elevation Profile

Intersect the continuation of the blue-blazed Riprap Trail at 0.4 mile. ▶2 Turn left as the Riprap Trail makes a sharp switchback to the right at 0.5 mile, then begin to descend, passing through a chestnut oak forest. A chestnut oak has thick leaves with wavy, rounded lobes on both sides of the leaf. Its acorns have been a primary food source for park animals since the demise of the chestnut tree in the early 1900s. Notice also a primary understory tree of the chestnut oak forest, the striped maple. The small tree is distinguished by its vertically striped bark and large, goosefoot-shaped leaves.

 Ridgeline

The Riprap Trail dips to a gap at 1.0 mile ▶3 and begins to climb, entering a rock field. Imagine the work involved in clearing the trail here and making it more foot-friendly. Achieve the crest of the ridge at 1.2 miles. ▶4 Immediately to your right is an outcrop with fine views into Paine Run below and the Shenandoah Valley beyond. Note the white quartz and the fascinating striations within. An old gnarled pine tree by the trail offers substantial shade for the hot hiker.

Continue heading west on the narrow ridge past a series of boulders. This is all part of aptly named Rocks Mountain. You reach the Calvary Rocks, a high knob on Rocks Mountain, at 1.4 miles. ▶5 Look for an old trail leading left to the top of the Calvary Rocks. The forest has reclaimed this outcrop, which offered views in days gone by. The park service used to cut back the vegetation as they do at Skyline Drive overlooks, but they stopped the practice after the area was designated a wilderness. Pass another lichen-covered boulder field. Look for ferns hiding in the moist, shady crevasses. Descend and then take the side trail leading right to Chimney Rock at mile 1.7. ▶6 A few steps later, emerge on a prominent quartz outcrop.

 Geological Interest

Carefully step out. No matter the season, you can find the perfect combination of sun and shade

 Great Views

to suit the temperature. Look below into the crevasse formerly spanned by a bridge. Now look out from left to right. First you can see the patchwork quilt of land that is the Shenandoah Valley and, beyond, the Alleghenies. Below, Paine Run cuts its way west to the South River, a tributary of the South Fork Shenandoah River. Trayfoot Mountain rises across Paine Run, which at 3,374 feet is the second-highest peak in Shenandoah's South District. Open, gray talus slopes tattoo the mountainside. Finally, to your right the Blue Ridge rises majestically. There is plenty to see from here, even without a bridge to Chimney Rock.

☀ MILESTONES

▶1	0.0	Riprap Parking Area at milepost 90.0
▶2	0.4	Left on Riprap Trail as AT leaves right
▶3	1.0	Gap
▶4	1.2	Vista
▶5	1.4	Left on old trail to Calvary Rocks
▶6	1.7	Chimney Rock

The winter sun *shines weakly on the Riprap Trail and adjacent embedded boulders.*

Turk Branch Loop

This loop traverses the park's most southerly and seemingly most forgotten reaches. Leave the crest of the Blue Ridge and descend along remote Turk Branch, passing old-home sites where Turk Branch meets the South Fork Moormans River. Head up the uppermost part of the rocky South Fork Moormans River valley to meet the Appalachian Trail (AT). Hike north on Shenandoah's master path, gaining limited views amid the pines and oaks before returning to Turk Gap. Though the elevation change is nearly 1,200 feet, the trail grades are never sharp.

Best Time

This is a good hike to take when other trails are busy, such as during summer and on holiday weekends. In springtime, you can enjoy streamside wildflowers and better view the trailside home sites. In fall, autumn colors show. You will find solitude year-round beyond the AT.

Finding the Trail

The Turk Gap Parking Area is located at milepost 94.1 on Skyline Drive, 10.5 miles north of the Rockfish Gap Entrance Station, on the east side of the drive.

Trail Description

The hardest part of this loop may be finding its beginning. Look for the concrete signpost directly beside Skyline Drive: here, the trail heads south

TRAIL USE
Day Hiking,
Backpacking
LENGTH
7.5 miles, 4–5 hours
VERTICAL FEET
±1,175'
DIFFICULTY
– 1 2 3 **4** 5 +
TRAIL TYPE
Loop
START & FINISH
N38° 07.751'
W78° 47.089'

FEATURES
Ridgeline
Stream
Waterfall
Autumn Colors
Wildflowers
Secluded
Historical Interest

FACILITIES
None

from the Turk Gap Parking Area. ▶1 Do *not* take the unmarked trail leaving from the end of the parking area farthest from Skyline Drive—make sure you're on the yellow-blazed Turk Branch Trail, and trace an old roadbed running parallel to Skyline Drive. Walk downhill through an oak-dominated forest. Skyline Drive rises to your right. At 0.3 mile, the Turk Branch Trail leads east, away from Skyline Drive. Descend on a dry ridgeline heavy with mountain laurel, scrub pines, and blueberries. Views of Bucks Elbow Mountain open between the trees.

Make a hard turn to the right at 1.0 mile. Descend to cross upper Turk Branch at 1.3 miles. ▶2 Black birch, maple, and cherry trees rise amid vines and ferns. Push over a rib ridge to cross a tributary of Turk Branch. Notice the stonework that has been done to level the old roadbed as it descends to cross Turk Branch again at 2.2 miles. ▶3 A low-flowing slab cascade drops above the Turk Branch crossing. Scant water keeps this fall modest and a lesser-visited destination.

The Turk Branch valley widens. White pines shade the trailside flats. Piled stones, rock walls, and leveled land indicate a homesite to the left of the trail. Meet the South Fork Moormans River Fire Road at 2.5 miles. ▶4 A survey marker has been embedded into a boulder at the junction. Turn right

Ridgeline ▲

Stream

Waterfall

Wildflowers

Turk Branch Loop Elevation Profile

Hikers see more snakes *in the South District than anywhere else in the park.*

here, and rock-hop Turk Branch under sycamores aplenty. Ascend to soon step over the South Fork Moormans River, which is but a small creek at this point. Watch for a few hemlocks that are hanging on. Pass a second homesite to the left of the trail, marked by rock walls, a clearing, a crumbling chimney, and metal relics. Please leave the remnants for others to discover and enjoy.

The grade steepens as the hollow narrows beyond the homesite. At 3.1 miles, cross South Fork Moormans River, then bisect a natural gas–line clearing. Step over what's left of the river one more time, and then intersect the AT at 4.3 miles, just below Jarman Gap. ▶5 Turn right here, hiking northbound on the AT. Dip along South Fork Moormans River one last time before ascending the east flank of the Blue Ridge, gaining views of Bucks Elbow Mountain across the Moormans River Valley. Climb more to cross the natural gas–line clearing at 5.0 miles. Top out on a piney knob at 5.4 miles. Windswept oaks and low-slung blueberries rise

Secluded

Historical
Interest

Ridgeline

from the slaty soil. Views soon open to the south and west as the AT levels. Sawmill Ridge and Turk Mountain stand in the distance.

Cross Skyline Drive and reach Sawmill Run Overlook at 6.0 miles. ▶6 Begin climbing beyond Skyline Drive. Curve right past a side trail leading left through tangled woods to a spring. Level off, then undulate along the path lined with blueberry bushes, mountain laurel, and sassafras (the last deciduous tree can be found throughout the Old Dominion and here, along the AT). The AT along this stretch of the Blue Ridge makes for pleasant hiking without extensive elevation changes.

Intersect the Turk Mountain Trail at 7.3 miles. ▶7 Keep north on the AT, and dip through some pines to emerge at Turk Gap at 7.5 miles, ending your loop. ▶8

𝆓	**MILESTONES**	
▶1	0.0	Turk Gap Parking Area at milepost 94.1
▶2	1.3	Cross Turk Branch
▶3	2.2	Cross Turk Branch, and pass a cascade
▶4	2.5	Right on South Fork Moormans River Fire Road
▶5	4.3	Right on the AT
▶6	6.0	Cross Skyline Drive at Sawmill Run Overlook
▶7	7.3	Turk Mountain Trail leaves left
▶8	7.5	Turk Gap Parking Area at milepost 94.1

The Appalachian Trail is a pleasant, level track in stretches.

Turk Mountain

Cool Spring Hollow

To Swift Run Gap

Turk Gap Trail

Skyline Drive

SHENANDOAH
NATIONAL
PARK

94
1

Turk Gap

Turk
Mountain

Turk Mountain Trail

Turk Branch Trail

Turk Branch

Skyline Drive

To Rockfish Gap

N

| 0 | 0.1 | 0.2 | 0.3 mile |
| 0 | 0.1 | 0.2 | 0.3 kilometer |

Turk Mountain

This was my first hike ever in Shenandoah National Park. Turk Mountain makes a great initiation hike for park visitors entering Shenandoah from the southern end. But no matter where you come from, you will not be disappointed by the outstanding views from the mountain's rocky summit.

Best Time

Hikers come here for the views and the rock outcrops. Anytime after cold fronts pass through or when it's clear is good.

Finding the Trail

The Turk Gap Parking Area is located at milepost 94.1 on the east side of Skyline Drive, 10.5 miles north of the Rockfish Gap Entrance Station.

Trail Description

Start your hike at Turk Gap. ▶1 Cross Skyline Drive and begin descending on the Appalachian Trail (AT), southbound. Immediately enter a stand of pines. Be sure to take the trail to the left once you cross the road. The trail to the right is the Turk Gap Trail. Walk under mountain laurel, maple, and chestnut oaks. Arrive at a trail junction at 0.2 mile. ▶2 Veer right on the lesser-used Turk Mountain Trail, descending to an unnamed gap at 0.5 mile. ▶3 Turk Mountain rises through the trees.

TRAIL USE
Day Hiking
LENGTH
2.4 miles, 2–2.5 hours
VERTICAL FEET
±500'
DIFFICULTY
– 1 **2** 3 4 5 +
TRAIL TYPE
Out-and-back
START & FINISH
N38° 07.751'
W78° 47.089'

FEATURES
Ridgeline
Summit
Autumn Colors
Great Views
Secluded
Geological Interest

FACILITIES
None

Ridgeline ▲

Autumn Colors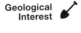

Geological Interest ✐

Summit △

Great Views 🔭

The trail climbs the rocky east slope of Turk Mountain cloaked in hickory–oak forest and soon enters a rock field. Continue through the rock field. The trail is rockier too.

The Turk Mountain Trail comes to a sharp right turn at 1.1 miles. ►4 You can scramble onto the rocks to your left for southerly views, but the big boulders are unstable and the views are better atop the summit. The trail continues to the right, then passes among some large boulders just before attaining the crest of the mountain.

At the crest, turn right to walk an irregular rock ridge, pocked with short trees that have gained purchase on thin soils. You make it to an elevated rock outcrop and the summit of Turk Mountain (2,981') at 1.2 miles. ►5 The views are outstanding. Below, a talus slope lays bare the mountainside, opening westerly views into Crimora and the Shenandoah Valley below. To your north rises wave upon wave of wooded mountains. On the far side of the valley are the Allegheny Mountains and the George Washington National Forest. Back to the east is Middle Mountain with its radio towers. To the south stands Calf Mountain, which is also growing radio towers. The talus slope itself is an exquisite jumble of whitish-gray broken rocks, resembling play blocks of mountain giants, upon which no human walks.

Turk Mountain Elevation Profile

Boulder-studded view *from Turk Mountain*

	MILESTONES	
▶1	0.0	Turk Gap Parking Area at milepost 94.1
▶2	0.2	Right on Turk Mountain Trail as AT leaves left
▶3	0.5	Gap
▶4	1.1	Right turn
▶5	1.2	Top of Turk Mountain with views

Appendix

Local Resources

National Park Service
Shenandoah National Park
540-999-3500, nps.gov/shen

The park's website has a wealth of information, including multimedia presentations about the park (nps.gov/shen/photosmultimedia/index.htm). If you can't find the information you desire on the website, then call the main park number and follow the prompts.

U.S. Forest Service
George Washington and Jefferson National Forests
888-265-0019, www.fs.usda.gov/gwj

Shenandoah visitors sometimes use the George Washington National Forest, which borders Shenandoah's south and west sides.

Shenandoah Partnership Groups
Shenandoah Valley Travel Association
800-847-4878, visitshenandoah.org

This website is your best portal for contacting the tourist bureaus of the greater Shenandoah Valley from top to bottom. Simply find your geographic area of interest, click on the link for that area, and look for the information you need.

Shenandoah National Park Association (SNPA)
540-999-3582, snpbooks.org

Established in 1950, the SNPA supports the interpretive and educational activities of Shenandoah National Park. Since its inception, the SNPA has donated more than $2 million to the park through its sales of books, maps, merchandise, and memorabilia. Check their website for a wealth of books and other sources of information about your Shenandoah area of interest.

Potomac Appalachian Trail Club (PATC)
703-242-0968, patc.net

The PATC is a large organization that helps maintain the Appalachian Trail and other trails throughout much of the Mid-Atlantic. They also maintain many trails within the Shenandoah National Park trail system. Within the park, they maintain backcountry huts and rental cabins. The PATC creates the primary trail maps used for Shenandoah's three districts, which are sold online and at park visitor centers. Joining the PATC is a great way to give your time, talent, and treasure to Shenandoah National Park.

Index

Note: Page numbers in **bold** represent photos.

About the Author

Photo: Keri Anne Molloy

Johnny Molloy is a writer and adventurer based in Johnson City, Tennessee. His passion for the outdoors started on a backpacking trip in Great Smoky Mountains National Park while he was attending the University of Tennessee. That first foray unleashed a love of the outdoors that led the Tennessee native to spend most of his time backpacking, canoe camping, and tent camping for the past three decades.

Friends enjoyed Johnny's outdoor adventure stories; one even suggested he write a book. He pursued his friend's idea and soon parlayed his love of the outdoors into an occupation. The results of his efforts are more than 60 books. His writings include hiking, camping, paddling, and comprehensive guidebooks about specific areas throughout the eastern United States, along with true-adventure guidebooks. He also writes for his local paper, the *Johnson City Press*, as well as for websites and magazines.

Johnny continues to write and travel extensively throughout the United States, endeavoring in a variety of outdoor pursuits. His nonoutdoor interests include American history, being a Gideon, and University of Tennessee sports. For more about Johnny, visit his website, johnnymolloy.com.